IMAGING OF THE ACUTELY ILL AND SURGICAL PATIENT

A Practical Guide

NOTICE

Medicine is an ever-changing science. As new research and clinical experience broaden our knowledge, changes in treatment and drug therapy are required. The authors and the publisher of this work have checked with sources believed to be reliable in their efforts to provide information that is complete and generally in accord with the standards accepted at the time of publication. However, in view of the possibility of human error or changes in medical sciences, neither the authors nor the publisher nor any other party who has been involved in the preparation or publication of this work warrants that the information contained herein is in every respect accurate or complete, and they disclaim all responsibility for any errors or omissions or for the results obtained from use of the information contained in this work. Readers are encouraged to confirm the information contained herein with other sources. For example and in particular, readers are advised to check the product information sheet included in the package of each drug they plan to administer to be certain that the information contained in this work is accurate and that changes have not been made in the recommended dose or in the contraindications for administration. This recommendation is of particular importance in connection with new or infrequently used drugs.

IMAGING OF THE ACUTELY ILL AND SURGICAL PATIENT

A Practical Guide

EDITORS

Bok Y. Lee, MD

Professor of Surgery
New York Medical College, Valhalla, New York

Director of Surgical Research
Sound Shore Medical Center, New Rochelle, New York

Adjunct Professor
Rensselaer Polytechnic Institute, Troy, New York

John H. Rundback, MD

Associate Professor of Radiology and Surgery
New York Medical College, Valhalla, New York

Director, Vascular and Interventional Radiology
Danbury Hospital, Danbury, Connecticut

Maurice R. Poplausky, MD

Assistant Professor of Radiology and Surgery, New York Medical College
Attending Physician, Vascular and Interventional Radiology
Westchester Medical Center, Valhalla, NY

McGraw-Hill
MEDICAL PUBLISHING DIVISION

New York / St. Louis / San Francisco / Auckland / Bogotá / Caracas / Lisbon
London / Madrid / Mexico City / Milan / Montreal / New Delhi
San Juan / Singapore / Sydney / Tokyo / Toronto

McGraw-Hill

A Division of The McGraw·Hill Companies

IMAGING OF THE ACUTELY ILL AND SURGICAL PATIENT:
A Practical Guide

1234567890 KGPKGP 01234567890

This book was set in Times Roman by York Graphic Services, Inc.
The editors were Michael Medina, Susan R. Noujaim, and Karen Davis.
The production supervisor was Catherine H. Saggese.
The cover designer was Aimeé Nordin.
The index was prepared by Angie Wiley.
Quebecor World/Kingsport was printer and binder.

This book is printed on acid-free paper.

ISBN   0-8385-4071-6

Library of Congress Cataloging-in-Publication Data

Imaging of the acutely ill and surgical patient: a practical guide / editors, Bok Y. Lee, John Rundback, Maurice R. Poplausky.
    p. ; cm.
    Includes bibliographical references and index.
    ISBN 0-8385-4071-6 (alk. paper)
    1. Diagnostic imaging—Atlases. 2. Interventional radiology—Atlases. 3. Surgery—Atlases. I. Lee, Bok Y., 1928- II. Rundback, John. III. Poplausky, Maurice R.
    [DNLM: 1. Diagnostic Imaging—methods—Atlases. 2. Acute Disease—Atlases. 3. Surgical Procedures, Operative—methods—Atlases. WN 17 I31 2001]
    RD33.55 .I435 2001
    616.07'54—dc21

00-020714

CONTENTS

Chapter 5
EXTREMITY IMAGING   133

Chapter 6
CATHETERS AND TUBES   153

CONTRIBUTORS

Adele Brudnicki, MD
Assistant Professor of Radiology
New York Medical College
Director, Pediatric Radiology
Westchester Medical Center

Gastone Crea, MD
Assistant Professor of Radiology
New York Medical College
Westchester Medical Center

Susan A. Klein, MD
Associate Professor of Radiology
New York Medical College
Director, Body Imaging
Director, Residency Program
Westchester Medical Center

Steven A. Kroop, MD
Assistant Professor of Radiology
New York Medical College
Associate Director, Nuclear Medicine
Westchester Medical Center

Shekher Maddineni, MD
Assistant Professor of Radiology
New York Medical College
Westchester Medical Center

Terence A.S. Matalon, MD
Professor and Chairman of Radiology
New York Medical College
Westchester Medical Center

Aria Parker, MD
Assistant Professor of Radiology
New York Medical College
Westchester Medical Center

Susan Rachlin, MD
Assistant Professor of Radiology
New York Medical College
Director, Medical Student Education
Associate Director, Residency Program
Westchester Medical Center

Alla Rozenblit, MD
Associate Professor of Radiology
Albert Einstein College of Medicine
Director, Body Imaging
Montefiore Medical Center

Grigory N. Rozenblit, MD
Associate Professor of Clinical Radiology
New York Medical College
Director, Vascular and Interventional Radiology
Westchester Medical Center

Michael H. Swirsky, MD
Associate Professor of Clinical Radiology
New York Medical College
Westchester Medical Center

Imre Weitzner Jr., MD
Assistant Professor of Radiology
New York Medical College
Westchester Medical Center

Joseph R. Zuback, DO
Assistant Professor of Radiology
New York Medical College
Westchester Medical Center

PREFACE

Physicians treating acutely ill patients are confronted daily with a vast array of diagnostic imaging modalities from which to choose. In the current environment of rapidly evolving image technology, it is increasingly important for surgical and medicine trainees and practitioners to appropriately utilize and properly interpret those images relevant to the diseases they treat. In addition, such images have recently been included on surgical and emergency medicine board examinations.

This book is intended as an informative and up-to-date atlas of representative radiologic images encountered in the evaluation of patients with surgical and acute medical conditions. Carefully selected and annotated images from multiple radiological modalities are provided, with an accompanying brief description of the disease process they represent. It is our goal that this "see-and-read" format will enhance the "pattern recognition" skills requisite for accurate radiologic diagnosis, and thus allow greater confidence for the surgical and emergency medicine trainee and practicing clinician who care for acutely ill and surgical patients.

John H. Rundback, MD
Maurice R. Poplausky, MD
Bok Y. Lee, MD

ACKNOWLEDGMENTS

We would like to acknowledge the contributions of the entire faculty of the New York Medical College Department of Radiology. We also acknowledge our clerical and technical staff for their help in preparing the manuscript and many of the images: Diane Forman, Suzanne Marigliano, Claudio Cantu, Lucy Osborne, and Billy Cleary. Last, but by no means least, we would like to thank our families, and particularly our wives Lili Rundback, Hannah Poplausky, and Taihee Lee for their patience and encouragement despite countless hours spent on the computer and sorting through pictures. The line artwork for this book comes from Bok Y. Lee. (1983). *Atlas of Surgical and Sectional Anatomy,* Appleton-Century-Crofts, East Norwalk, Connecticut.

CHAPTER 1

NEURORADIOLOGY

Maurice R. Poplausky, MD

John H. Rundback, MD

Bok Y. Lee, MD, FACS

1.1 NORMALS

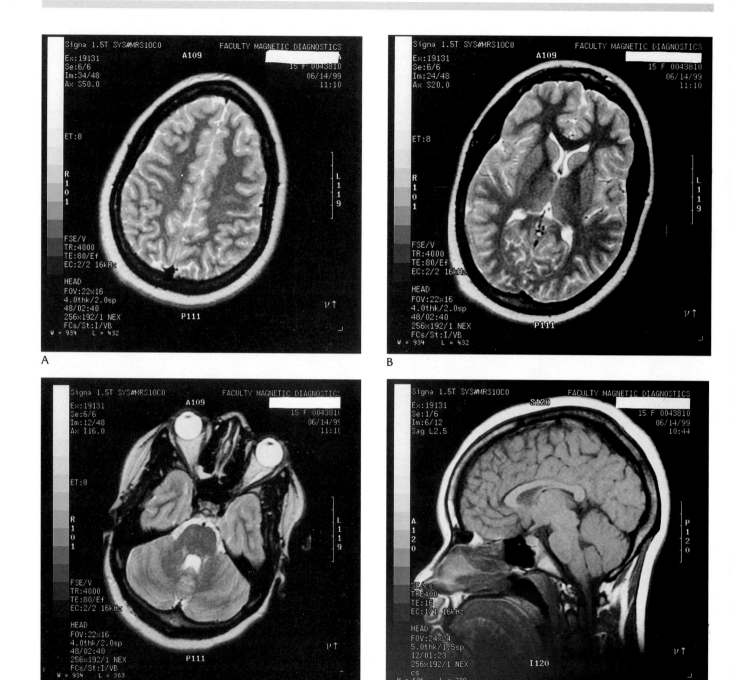

Figure 1–1A–D Normal MRI scans of the brain at a level above the ventricles (**A**), see opposite page, through the lateral ventricles (**B**), see page 4, and at the posterior fossa and skull base (**C**), see page 5. A sagittal MRI (**D**) shows normal midline structures. MRI has the advantage of multiplanar imaging.

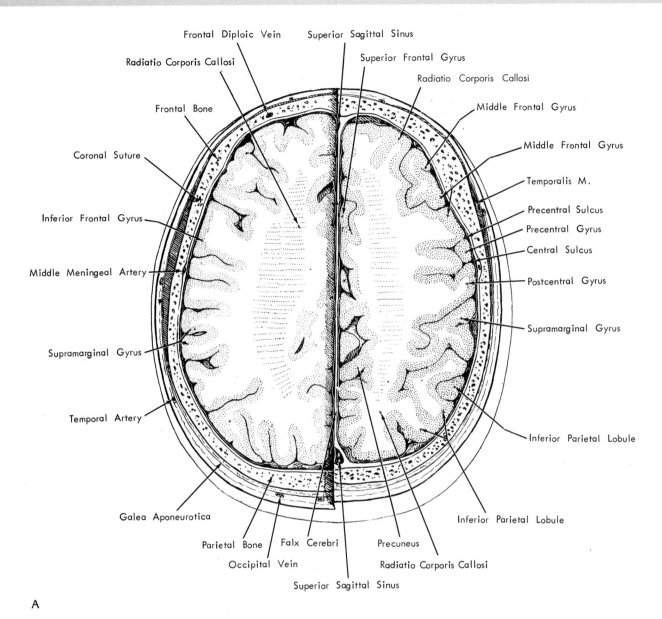

A

Figure 1–2A–C Line drawings corresponding to Figures 1–1A–C, show normal brain anatomy.

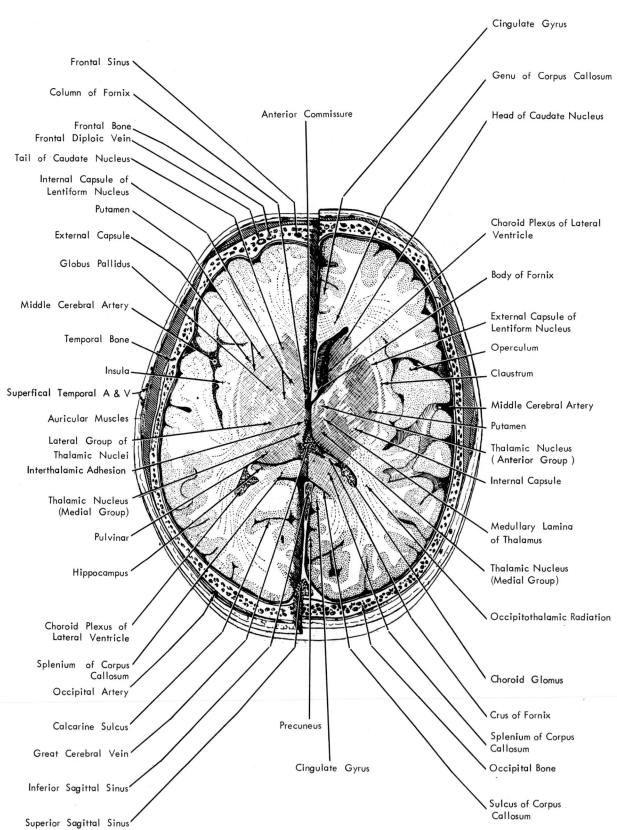

Cingulate Gyrus

Genu of Corpus Callosum

Head of Caudate Nucleus

Frontal Sinus

Column of Fornix

Frontal Bone
Frontal Diploic Vein

Tail of Caudate Nucleus

Internal Capsule of
Lentiform Nucleus

Putamen

External Capsule

Globus Pallidus

Middle Cerebral Artery

Temporal Bone

Insula

Superfical Temporal A & V

Auricular Muscles

Lateral Group of
Thalamic Nuclei

Interthalamic Adhesion

Thalamic Nucleus
(Medial Group)

Pulvinar

Hippocampus

Choroid Plexus of
Lateral Ventricle

Splenium of Corpus
Callosum

Occipital Artery

Calcarine Sulcus

Great Cerebral Vein

Inferior Sagittal Sinus

Superior Sagittal Sinus

Anterior Commissure

Precuneus

Cingulate Gyrus

Choroid Plexus of Lateral
Ventricle

Body of Fornix

External Capsule of
Lentiform Nucleus

Operculum

Claustrum

Middle Cerebral Artery

Putamen

Thalamic Nucleus
(Anterior Group)

Internal Capsule

Medullary Lamina
of Thalamus

Thalamic Nucleus
(Medial Group)

Occipitothalamic Radiation

Choroid Glomus

Crus of Fornix

Splenium of Corpus
Callosum

Occipital Bone

Sulcus of Corpus
Callosum

B

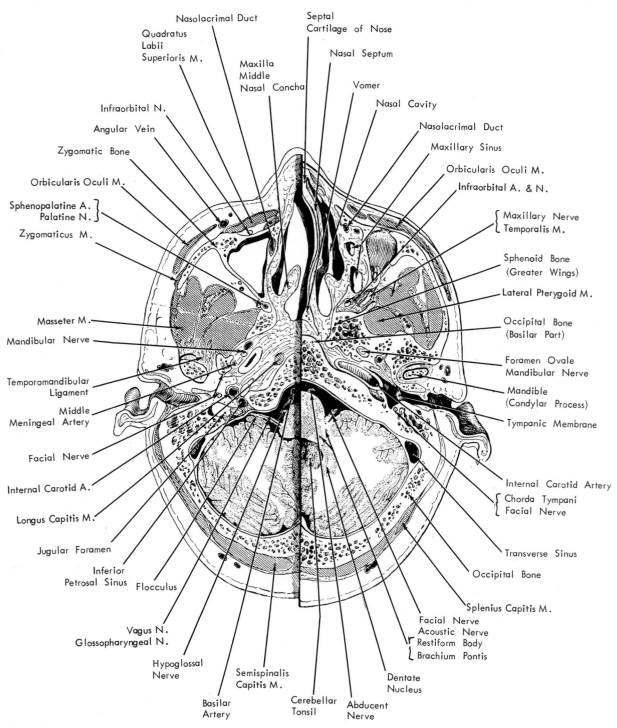

Nasolacrimal Duct

Quadratus Labii Superioris M.

Maxilla Middle Nasal Concha

Septal Cartilage of Nose

Nasal Septum

Vomer

Nasal Cavity

Infraorbital N.

Angular Vein

Zygomatic Bone

Orbicularis Oculi M.

Sphenopalatine A. Palatine N.

Zygomaticus M.

Masseter M.

Mandibular Nerve

Temporomandibular Ligament

Middle Meningeal Artery

Facial Nerve

Internal Carotid A.

Longus Capitis M.

Jugular Foramen

Inferior Petrosal Sinus

Flocculus

Vagus N.
Glossopharyngeal N.

Hypoglossal Nerve

Basilar Artery

Semispinalis Capitis M.

Cerebellar Tonsil

Abducent Nerve

Dentate Nucleus

Facial Nerve
Acoustic Nerve
Restiform Body
Brachium Pontis

Splenius Capitis M.

Occipital Bone

Transverse Sinus

Internal Carotid Artery

Chorda Tympani
Facial Nerve

Tympanic Membrane

Mandible (Condylar Process)

Foramen Ovale
Mandibular Nerve

Occipital Bone (Basilar Part)

Lateral Pterygoid M.

Sphenoid Bone (Greater Wings)

Maxillary Nerve
Temporalis M.

Infraorbital A. & N.

Orbicularis Oculi M.

Maxillary Sinus

Nasolacrimal Duct

C

1.2 CEREBRAL INFARCTION

Cerebral infarction, also referred to as a stroke, cerebrovascular accident (CVA), or brain attack, affects over 700,000 persons yearly in the United States resulting in over 150,000 deaths. Stroke is the leading cause of adult disability and the third leading cause of death in the United States. Nearly 75% of strokes occur because of occlusion of the intracranial vessels by emboli arising from atherosclerotic plaque at the cervical carotid bifurcation. In both asymptomatic and symptomatic patients with carotid stenosis >70%, carotid endarterectomy has proved efficacious in reducing the incidence of strokes when compared with medical therapy alone. The recent development of percutaneous stenting of the carotid arteries appears to show similar promise as a means of preventing strokes in patients with extracranial carotid disease. Carotid stenosis is most commonly diagnosed using duplex sonography, with both spectral velocities and imaging appearance used to measure lesion severity. Magnetic resonance angiography (MRA) may also be used, particularly for patients also requiring intracranial evaluation. Angiography is the gold standard for diagnosis, and is used for clarifying those cases in which patients have equivocal stenoses on other imaging modalities as well as prior to surgical or percutaneous revascularization.

The mainstay for imaging of strokes is computed tomography (CT). While a nonhemorrhagic event may not be visible on a CT scan within the first 8 to 24 hours after the neurologic event, potential early findings include the hyperdense middle cerebral artery sign (signifying arterial thrombosis) and the absence of filling of cortical veins in the affected hemisphere. In contrast, hemorrhagic infarcts are readily apparent by the pres-ence of hyperdense blood within the brain parenchyma. In the subacute phase, CT will show a hypodense wedge-shaped lesion, mass effect owing to white matter edema, loss of gray–white matter differentiation, and effacement of the cortical sulci in the affected region. Chronic infarcts, on the other hand, result in loss of volume and the accompanying enlargement of the sulci and the ipsilateral ventricle.

Magnetic resonance imaging (MRI) will depict an acute nonhemorrhagic stroke earlier than CT, with abnormalities becoming apparent within 1 to 6 hours after the event. Early findings include low-signal intensity of the affected region on T_1-weighted images, high-signal intensity on T_2-weighted images, and loss of the signal void within cortical veins. Intravenous or catheter-directed thrombolysis is currently under intensive investigation, and may reduce the extent of cerebral injury in selected cases, albeit at the risk of developing intracranial bleeding.

SELECTED REFERENCES

Bahn MM, Oser AB, Cross DT III. CT and MRI of stroke. J Magn Reson Imaging. 1996; 6: 833–845.

Maeda M, Abe H, Yamada H, Ishii Y. Hyperacute infarction: a comparison of CT and MRI, including diffusion-weighted imaging. Neuroradiology. 1999; 41: 175–178.

Baird AE, Warach S. Magnetic resonance imaging of acute stroke. J Cereb Blood Flow Metab. 1998; 18: 583–609.

Alberts MJ. Hyperacute stroke therapy with tissue plasminogen activator. Am J Cardiol. 1997; 80: 29D–34D.

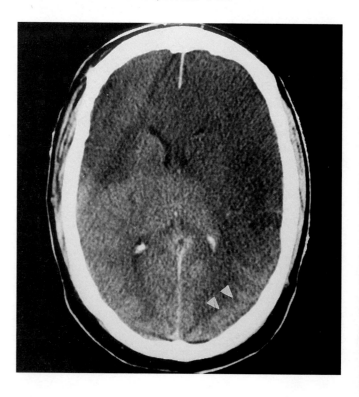

Figure 1–3 Cerebral infarction. A noncontrast CT scan of the brain at the level of the frontal horns reveals diffuse low attenuation in the distribution of the right anterior cerebral artery (representing a frontal infarction) as well as left anterior and middle cerebral arteries (representing a frontoparietal infarction). There is loss of the normal gray–white junction in the infarcted areas. In contrast, the gray–white junction is preserved in the occipital region (arrowheads).

1.3 BERRY ANEURYSM/SUBARACHNOID HEMORRHAGE

While bleeding into the subarachnoid space can occur as a sequela of trauma, the most common and classic cause is rupture of a congenital "berry" aneurysm. Intracerebral aneurysms occur in 1–10% of the American population, with 95% of aneurysms found in the vascular distribution of the internal carotid artery. Typical aneurysm sites are the anterior communicating artery in 30–35%, the internal carotid or posterior communicating artery in 30–35%, the middle cerebral artery bifurcation in 20%, and the posterior circulation in 10%. All patients with subarachnoid hemorrhage (SAH) should undergo a complete 4-vessel cerebral angiogram as multiple aneurysms are present in 20–25% of cases. There is a 1–2%/year risk of rupture if left untreated.

A noncontrast CT examination should be performed first for the evaluation of SAH, which will appear as high-attenuation material (blood) in the cerebral sulci and basal cisterns. Although sometimes subtle, communicating hydrocephalus is almost always present. A contrast-enhanced CT can occasionally show an aneurysm as a collection of contrast adjacent to a vessel. MRI is not a sensitive modality for diagnosing SAH, although MRA reliably reveals underlying vascular disease.

Neurosurgical clipping has been the standard of practice for treating intracranial aneurysms. At specialized centers during the past several years, aneurysms have been successfully treated with catheter-directed embolization of the aneurysm sac or feeding artery using detachable coils.

SELECTED REFERENCES

Harrison MJ, Johnson BA, Gardner GM, Welling BG. Preliminary results on the management of unruptured intracranial aneurysms with magnetic resonance angiography and computed tomographic angiography. Neurosurgery. 1997; 40: 947–955.

Young BJ, Seigerman MH, Hurst RW. Subarachnoid hemorrhage and aneurysms. Semin Ultrasound CT MR. 1996; 17: 265–277.

Vieco PT, Shuman WP, Alsofrom GF, Gross CE. Detection of circle of Willis aneurysms in patients with acute subarachnoid hemorrhage: a comparison of CT angiography and digital subtraction angiography. AJR 1995; 165: 425–430.

Atlas SW. Magnetic resonance imaging of intracranial aneurysms. Neuroimaging Clin North Am. 1997; 7: 709–720.

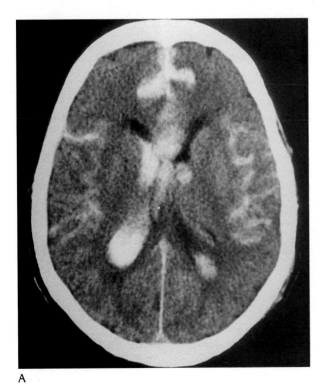
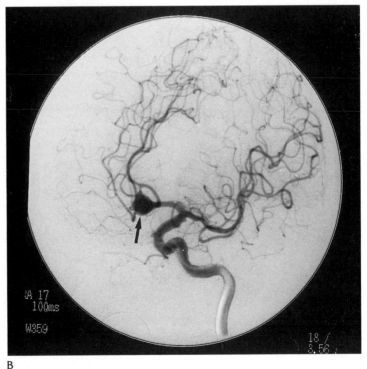

A   B

Figure 1–4A–B Subarachnoid hemorrhage.   A noncontrast CT scan (**A**) shows high-density blood within the lateral ventricles and outlining the cerebral sulci. A cerebral arteriogram on the same patient (**B**) reveals a large fusiform aneurysm of the anterior communicating artery (arrow), the most common site for intracranial aneurysms.

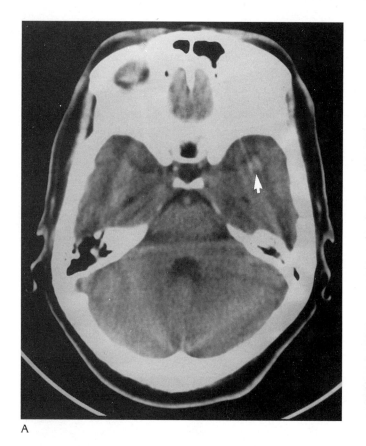

A

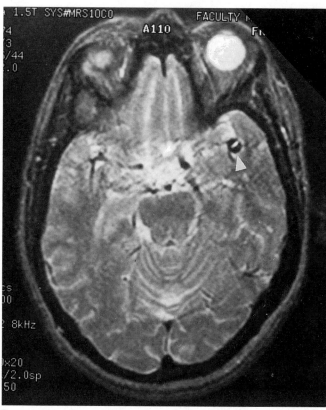

B

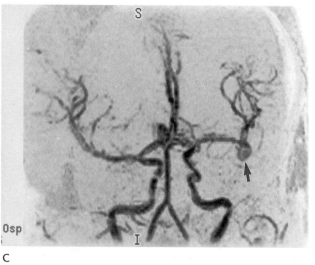

C

Figure 1–5A–C Middle cerebral artery aneurysm. On an enhanced CT scan of the brain (**A**), a focal dilatation of the left middle cerebral artery is noted (arrow). A corresponding magnetic resonance scan (**B**) shows a "signal void" at the same location (arrowhead). The magnetic resonance angiogram on the same patient (**C**) clearly depicts the aneurysm at the middle cerebral artery bifurcation (black arrow).

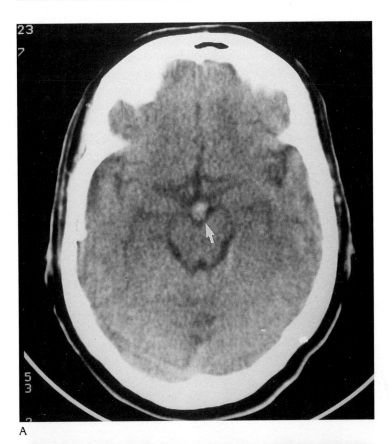

A

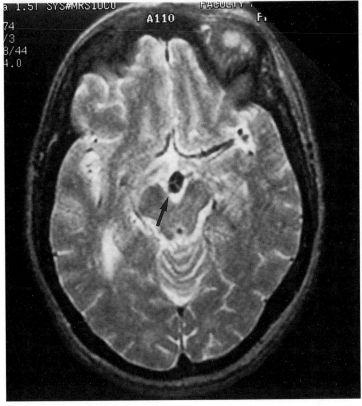

B

Figure 1–6A, B Basilar tip aneurysm. A CT scan (**A**) and MRI (**B**) show a characteristic aneurysm of the top of the basilar artery (arrows).

1.4 SUBDURAL HEMATOMA

Subdural hematomas (SDHs) almost always occur as a result of trauma due to stretching and tearing of bridging dural veins. SDHs are classified as acute when identified within the first 72 hours, subacute when recognized between 3 and 20 days, and chronic when more than 20 days old. CT and MR findings depend on the age of the lesion. On cross-sectional imaging, SDHs are crescent-shaped extracerebral collections of blood, most commonly occurring over the frontal or parietal convexity of the brain, and less often seen along the free edge of the falx cerebri or tentorium cerebelli. Acute subdural hematomas appear as high-attenuation lesions on CT, and can be associated with midline shift and effacement of the sulci when the SDHs are large. Subacute subdural hematomas become isodense with the brain, and are thus much more difficult to detect on CT, although contrast-enhanced scans will show displacement of the cortical vessels away from the calvarium by the SDH. Chronic subdural hematomas are low-attenuation crescent-shaped lesions.

On MRI, acute subdural hematomas are isointense on T_1-weighted images and hypointense on T_2-weighted images. Subacute subdural hematomas become much easier to see on MR imaging because of the ferromagnetic properties of methemoglobin, and T_1-weighted images show the hematoma as hyperintense relative to the brain parenchyma. Chronic SDHs usually appear as high signal lesions on both T_1 and T_2 sequences, although up to 30% may be iso- to hypointense. Up to 50% of patients who present with chronic SDHs are chronic alcoholics.

SELECTED REFERENCES

Johnson MH, Lee SH. Computed tomography of acute cerebral trauma. Radiol Clin North Am. 1992; 30: 325–352.

Wilms G, Marachal G, Geusens E, et al. Isodense subdural haematomas on CT: MRI findings. Neuroradiology. 1992; 34: 497–499.

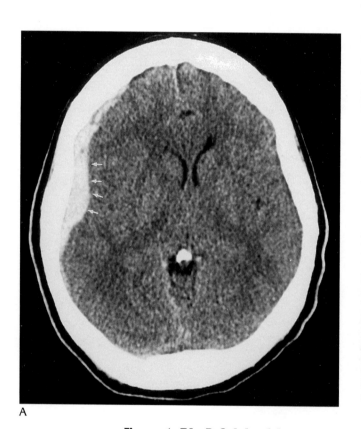

A

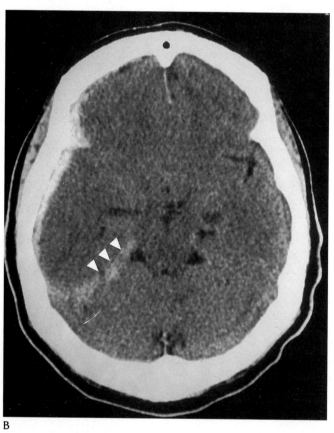

B

Figure 1–7A, B Subdural hematoma. A concave right frontoparietal collection of blood is present on a noncontrast CT scan (**A**). Blood along the free edge of the tentorium is noted (**B**, arrowheads).

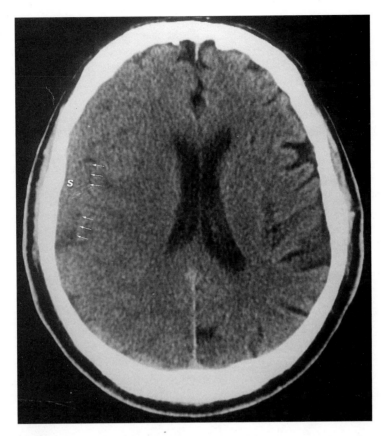

Figure 1–8 Isodense subdural hematoma. Subacute hematomas have the same density as the normal adjacent brain parenchyma. Effacement of the cerebral sulci on the affected side (small arrows) is the only evidence of the collection. In comparison, the sulci on the left are preserved.

1.5 EPIDURAL HEMATOMA AND ABSCESS

Epidural hematomas are collections of blood between the inner table of the skull and the dura, caused by a laceration of the meningeal artery or vein on the calvarial surface. Epidural hematomas are one-tenth as common as subdural hematomas, rarely occur in patients younger than 2 years of age or older than 60 years of age, and are associated with skull fractures in >80% of cases. Superimposed infection may result in epidural abscess formation. However, pyogenic infection of the epidural space is more commonly seen as a sequela of complicated paranasal sinusitis.

Acute epidural collections appear on CT as high-attenuation biconvex lesions adjacent to the skull. Mass effect is commonly seen, although underlying brain injury is uncommon. Since the blood collects in the space between the dura and the inner table of the skull, epidural hematomas do not cross suture lines (lo-cations where the dura is firmly attached to the skull). On MR, the shape is the same as that described for CT with signal characterisics related to the age of the hematoma. Epidural empyemas are uncommon and will appear as gas-fluid levels on CT. Urgent neurosurgical evacuation of epidural lesions is critical.

SELECTED REFERENCES

Teasdale G, Teasdale E, Hadley D. Computed tomographic and magnetic resonance imaging classification of head injury. J Neurotrauma. 1992; 1: S249–S257.

Gallagher RM, Gross CW, Phillips CD. Suppurative intracranial complications of sinusitis. Laryngoscope. 1998; 108(11 pt 1): 1635–1642.

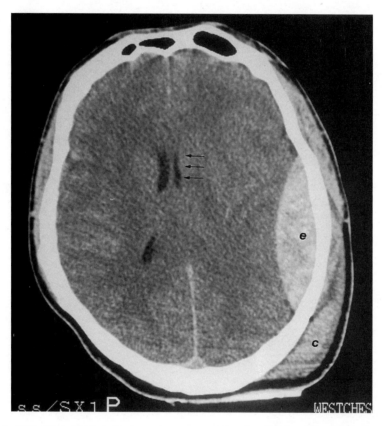

Figure 1–9 Epidural hematoma. An acute epidural collection (**e**) of blood assumes a high-attenuation biconvex (elliptical) configuration on a nonenhanced CT scan. An associated cephalohematoma (**c**) and compression of the left lateral ventricle (arrows) is also seen.

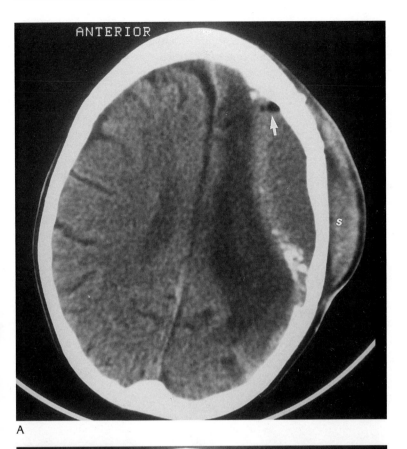

A

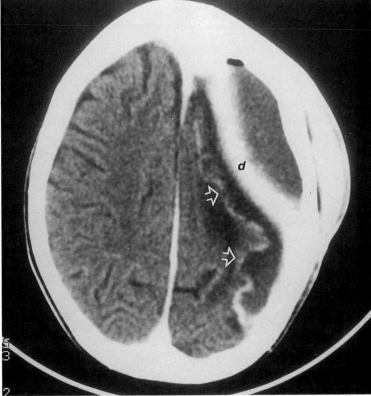

B

Figure 1–10A, B Epidural abscess. Nonenhanced (**A**) and contrast-enhanced (**B**) CT scans of the brain of a patient with a chronic posttraumatic epidural hematoma. The hematoma is isodense with the brain. Superimposed infection is manifested by air within the collection (arrow), soft tissue swelling (**s**), and marked enhancement of the adjacent pachymeninges (open arrows) and dura (**d**).

1.6 CEREBRAL CONTUSION

Cerebral contusions are posttraumatic lesions that histologically represent hemorrhage, necrosis, and edema. These "brain bruises" are predominantly cortical lesions, but when severe can involve the white matter. Contusions occur most commonly in the inferior aspect of the temporal and frontal lobes because of deceleration forces, when the "fluid" brain rubs against the fixed bony protuberances of the base of the skull. Bleeding may also develop at a site distant from the point of impact and is called a contrecoup lesion.

CT and MRI are the best modalities for evaluating brain contusions. On CT, varying amounts of high-attenuation material (representing blood) surrounded by low-attenuation regions (representing edema) are seen. Delayed hemorrhage can occur up to 48 hours after the initial insult in up to 20% of cases. If lesions are severe enough, mass affect can be seen, which peaks approximately 1 week after trauma. MRI reveals contusions well because the signal varies according to the age of the blood within the lesion. The surrounding edema always appears as high-signal areas on T_2-weighted images.

SELECTED REFERENCES

Yamaki T, Kirakawa K, Ueguchi T, et al. Chronological evaluation of acute traumatic intracerebral haematoma. Acta Neurochir (Wien). 1990; 1030: 112–115.

Bullock R, Maxwell WL, Graham DI, et al. Glial swelling following human cerebral contusion: an ultrastructural study. J Neurol Neurosurg Psychiatry. 1991; 54: 427–434.

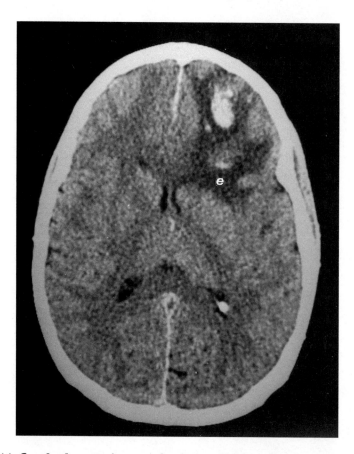

Figure 1–11 Cerebral contusion. A focal area of high attenuation representing acute intraparenchymal blood is seen in the left frontal lobe. There is surrounding low-attenuation white matter edema (**e**).

1.7 DIFFUSE AXONAL INJURY

As a result of differences in fluid characteristics, rotational or acceleration forces may produce shear injuries at the gray–white matter junction, and are called diffuse axonal injury. Axonal shear injuries occur in approximately 40% of patients with severe head trauma. It occurs most commonly in the frontal and temporal lobe white matter at the gray–white junction, the corpus callosum, and the dorsolateral aspect of the brain stem.

MRI is the best modality for evaluating axonal injury because of its superiority in detecting white matter disease. High-signal lesions are typically seen in the white matter on T_2-weighted images, and focal areas of hemorrhage can be seen. CT scans often show multifocal cerebral hemorrhages at the gray–white interface, although CT scans are not very sensitive when hemorrhage is not present. When a trauma patient presents with a low score on the Glasgow Coma Scale and a near-normal–appearing CT scan, diffuse axonal injury is most likely present. Delayed scans (days) are preferred and will eventually show the extent of the injury.

SELECTED REFERENCES

Sklar EM, Quencer RM, Bowen BC, et al. Magnetic resonance applications in cerebral injury. Radiol Clin North Am 1992; 30: 353–366.

Yokota H, Kurokawa A, Otsuka T, et al. Significance of magnetic resonance imaging in acute head injury. J Trauma. 1991; 31: 351–357.

Tomei G, Sganzerla E, Spagnoli D, et al. Posttraumatic diffuse cerebral lesions. Relationship between clinical course, CT findings and ICP. J Neurosurg Sci. 1991; 35: 61–75.

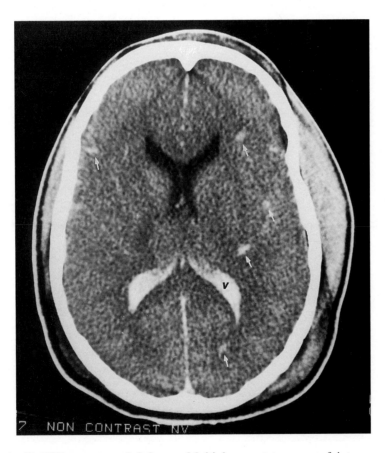

Figure 1–12 Diffuse axonal injury. Multiple punctate areas of intraparenchymal hemorrhage are seen (arrows). Blood is also layering in the occipital horns of both lateral ventricles (**v**).

1.8 ARTERIOVENOUS MALFORMATION

Cerebral arteriovenous malformations (AVMs) are developmental anomalies of the blood vessels in which cerebral arteries are in direct communication with draining veins without an intervening capillary network. AVMs occur in approximately 0.1% of the population, and are most often found in the parietal lobe. Fifty percent of patients present with intraparenchymal or subarachnoid hemorrhage, and an additional one third of patients present with a seizure disorder.

CT, MR, and angiography are the modalities of choice when evaluating AVMs. On nonenhanced CT scans, a mixed high- and low-attenuation lesion is seen that frequently contains calcifications. Some degree of local atrophy is always present. Contrast-enhanced CT scans show enhancing serpiginous tubular structures that represent the abnormal blood vessels. MRI displays flow void within the serpiginous vessels. An an-

giogram reveals an abnormal tangle of vessels with abnormally large feeding arteries and the early appearance of draining veins. In selected cases, transcatheter embolization of the feeding vessels and vascular nidus is possible. Other treatments include narrow-beam gamma-knife radiotherapy and neurosurgical excision of the vascular nidus.

SELECTED REFERENCES

Graves VB, Duff TA. Intracranial arteriovenous malformations. Current imaging and treatment. Invest Radiol. 1990; 25: 952–960.

Deveikis JP. Endovascular therapy of intracranial arteriovenous malformations. Materials and techniques. Neuroimaging Clin North Am. 1998; 8: 401–424.

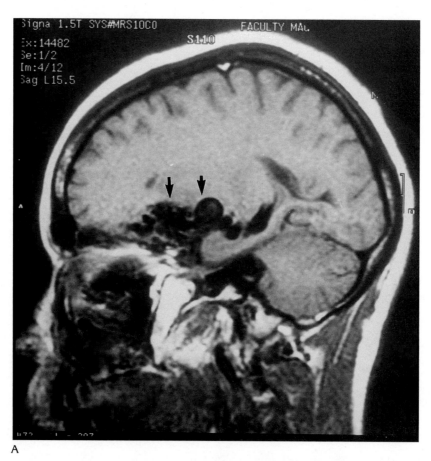

A

Figure 1–13A–C Arteriovenous malformation (AVM). A parasagittal T_1-weighted image (**A**) shows multiple serpiginous low-signal flow voids within the temporal lobe (arrows), diagnostic of an AVM. A 3-D–reconstructed CT angiogram (**B**) at the skull base again shows the dilated vascular structures including an enlarged vein (**v**) draining the lesion. Contrast angiography (**C**) of the same patient confirms the presence of an AVM.

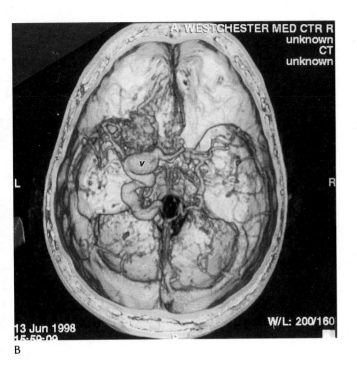

B

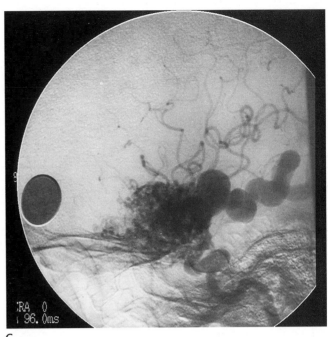

C

1.9 BRAIN ABSCESS

A brain abscess is an encapsulated purulent collection within the brain parenchyma, occurring as a result of trauma, meningitis, bacteremia, or direct extension from the sinuses or middle ear due to retrograde thrombophlebitis. Varying amounts of necrosis are present. When infection and inflammation occur without associated necrosis, the term cerebritis is used to describe the process. Abscesses generally occur in the white matter of the brain near the gray–white junction, may be single or multiple, and occur most commonly in the cerebral hemispheres. The following stages in abscess development have been described: early cerebritis (3 to 5 days), late cerebritis (4 to 5 days and as long as 10 to 14 days), early capsule (beginning at approximately 2 weeks), and late capsule (lasting weeks to months). Aerobic and anaerobic streptococcal infections are the most common organisms isolated; anaerobic infections predominate in adults. In children, abscesses are usually the result of staphylococcal or streptococcal pneumonia. Other pathogenic species seen in immunocompromised patients include Enterobacteriaceae, *Pseudomonas*, fungi, and mycobacteria.

CT and MRI are useful in diagnosing brain abscesses. In early lesions, postcontrast CT and MRI show enhancement in the region of infection with large amounts of surrounding vasogenic edema. As the lesion progresses, central necrosis occurs and an abscess wall develops after approximately 2 weeks. The abscess wall appears on CT as a smooth-walled ring of contrast enhancement, often thinner along the medial margin because of gray–white perfusion variation. The differential of a ring-enhancing lesion on CT includes: abscess, primary glioblastoma, or metastasis. The only finding on CT that is pathognomonic for brain abscess is gas within the central cavity. Treatment for most mature abscesses is surgical, although cerebritis and some abscesses may be treated with a prolonged course of parenteral antibiotics.

SELECTED REFERENCES

Mathisen GE, Johnson JP. Brain abscess. Clin Infect Dis. 1997; 25: 763–779.

Brook I. Brain abscess in children: microbiology and management. J Child Neurol. 1995; 10: 283–288.

Osenbach RK, Loftus CM. Diagnosis and management of brain abscess. Neurosurg Clin North Am. 1992; 3: 403–420.

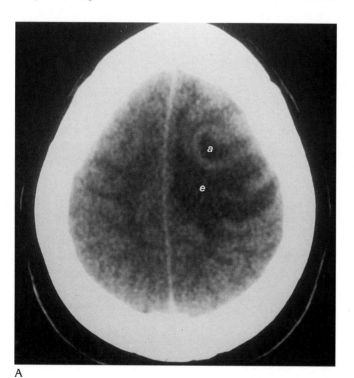

A

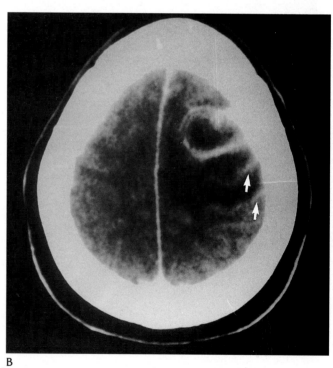

B

Figure 1–14A, B Brain abscess. A nonenhanced CT scan (**A**) shows a focal round low attenuation lesion (**a**) within the left frontoparietal lobe with surrounding vasogenic edema (**e**). A postcontrast scan (**B**) shows enhancement of the abscess wall and the adjacent meningeal surface (arrows).

1.10 MENINGITIS

Meningitis is the most common presentation of pyogenic infection in the central nervous system, and represents inflammation of the dural membranes and cerebral spinal fluid (CSF). Meningitis is most often the result of hematogenous spread of infection; other causes include trauma, direct extension from the sinuses, or as a sequela of a cerebral abscess. The offending organism is age-specific with *Escherichia coli* and group B streptococci being the most common in neonates, *Haemophilus influenzae* infection in infants and young children, and *Nisseria meningitides* and *Streptococcus pneumoniae* in patients older than 5 years old.

Meningitis is best diagnosed by lumbar puncture. Contrast-enhanced CT and MRI may show meningeal enhancement, predominantly at the base of the brain. Complications seen on CT include infarction (caused by cerebral vasospasm), hydro-cephalus (due to obstruction of the arachnoid granulations), subdural effusions or empyema, cerebritis or cerebral abscess formation, and ventriculitis.

SELECTED REFERENCES

Chang KH, Han MH, Roh JK, et al. Gd-DTPA-enhanced MR imaging of the brain in patients with meningitis: comparison with CT. AJR. 1990; 154: 809–816.

Runge VM, Wells JW, Williams NM, et al. Detectability of early brain meningitis with magnetic resonance imaging. Invest Radiol. 1995; 154: 484–495.

Kioumehr F, Dadsetan MR, Feldman N, et al. Postcontrast MRI of cranial meninges: leptomeningitis versus pachymeningitis. J Comput Assist Tomogr. 1995; 19: 713–720.

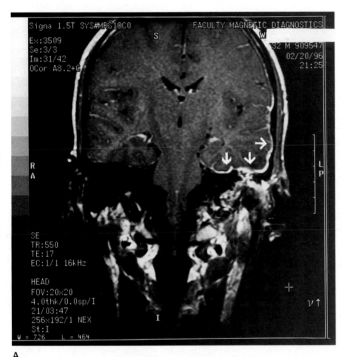

A

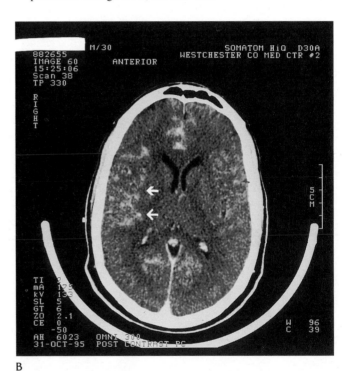

B

Figure 1–15A, B Meningitis. A coronal gadolinium-enhanced MR image of the brain (**A**) and postcontrast axial CT scan (**B**) of two different patients show asymmetric meningeal enhancement at the site of meningeal inflammation (arrows).

1.11 CEREBRAL NEOPLASMS

Tumors of the brain and the meninges account for approximately 9% of all neoplasms. Gliomas, metastases, meningiomas, pituitary adenomas, and acoustic neurinomas account for approximately 95% of all neoplasms occurring in the brain. Certain brain tumors have strong predilections for particular intracranial regions. Furthermore, particular types of tumors characteristically occur within a specific age range.

MRI, CT, and angiography are the principal diagnostic modalities used for evaluation of brain lesions. MRI is the most sensitive method for detecting tumors. Tumors appear as low signal on T_1-weighted images and as high signal on T_2-weighted images because of their high water content. Differentiation of tumor and edema could be difficult without the use of gadolinium enhancement. Following gadolinium administration, the neoplasm will usually become hyperintense on T_1-weighted images.

Contrast-enhanced CT is also effective in diagnosing intracranial neoplasms. Most tumors show contrast enhancement because of disruption to the blood–brain barrier. This disruption is seen as an area of increased attenuation, usually surrounded by an area of low attenuation that represents edema. Depending on the size and location of the neoplasm, a varying degree of mass affect and midline shift can be seen with both CT and MRI.

Angiography is no longer used as a primary diagnosing modality for brain tumors since the advent of CT and MRI. It is, however, used to help differentiate particular types of tumors and to determine their blood supply before intervention or surgery.

SELECTED REFERENCES

Sotaniemi KA, Rantala M, Pyhtinen J, Myllyla VV. Clinical and CT correlates in the diagnosis of intracranial tumours. J Neurol Neurosurg Psychiatry. 1991; 54: 645–647.

Allcutt DA, Mendelow AD. Presentation and diagnosis of brain tumours. Br J Hosp Med. 1992; 47: 745–752.

Go KG, Kamman RL, Pruim J, et al. On the principles underlying the diagnosis of brain tumours—a survey article. Acta Neurochir (Wien). 1995; 135: 1–11.

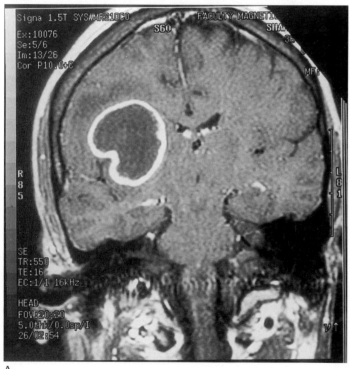

A

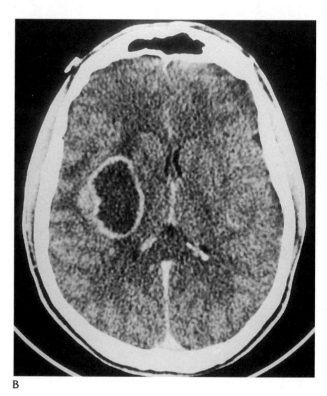

B

Figure 1–16A, B Brain neoplasm. A coronal gadolinium-enhanced MRI (**A**) shows a well-circumscribed right parietal lobe mass with enhancing walls and surrounding edema. A corresponding axial CT scan (**B**) again shows the low-attenuation mass with enhancing walls and surrounding edema.

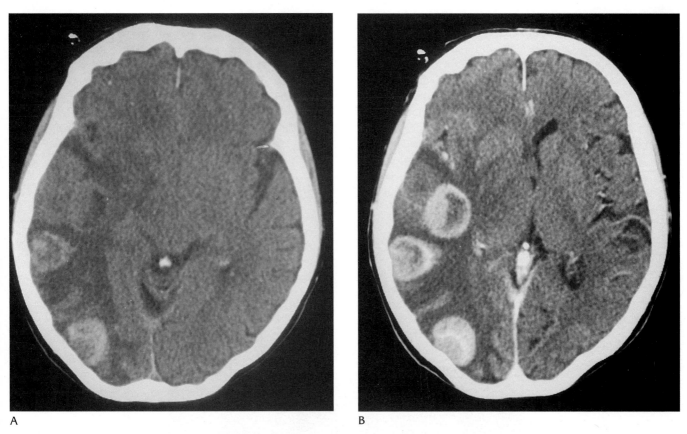

A

B

Figure 1–17A, B Brain metastases. Multiple nodules with surrounding edema are present in the right parieto-occipital lobe of this patient with metastatic breast carcinoma. The high attenuation of the lesions on the nonenhanced scan (**A**) represents hemorrhage. The lesions are ring-enhancing and more clearly delineated on a CT obtained after the administration of IV contrast (**B**).

1.12 HYDROCEPHALUS

Cerebral spinal fluid (CSF) is produced by the choroid plexus, which lines the ventricles, and then flows through the ventricular system to eventually exit the 4th ventricle through the foramina of Lushka and Magendi. CSF is then reabsorbed by the arachnoid granulations along the cerebral convexity. Hydrocephalus is the pathologic dilatation of the ventricular system usually caused by an obstruction within the normal pathway of CSF flow, and may involve all or part of the ventricular system (lateral horns, temporal horns, occipital horns, 3rd ventricle, and 4th ventricle). An obstruction anywhere along this route will cause hydrocephalus. Overproduction of CSF as a cause of hydrocephalus is rare, and is usually the result of a choroid plexus papilloma.

Obstructive hydrocephalus is further classified as being either a communicating or noncommunicating type. Communicating hydrocephalus is the most common type found in adults, and is caused by reduced reabsorption of CSF by the arachnoid granulations. This finding is commonly seen with subarachnoid hemorrhages. Noncommunicating hydrocephalus is caused by an obstruction of CSF flow in the ventricles or at the outlet foramina of the 4th ventricle. An intracerebral mass lesion or congenital narrowing is most commonly responsible for this type of hydrocephalus.

The diagnosis of hydrocephalus is best made with CT or MRI. Enlargement of part or all of the ventricular system is seen. A decrease in the size of sulci can also be seen because of compression by the expanded CSF space. Periventricular white matter edema may also occur, representing transependymal migration of the CSF.

SELECTED REFERENCES

Bradley WG Jr, Scalzo D, Queralt J, et al. Normal-pressure hydrocephalus: evaluation with cerebrospinal fluid flow measurements at MR imaging. Radiology. 1996; 198: 523–529.

Feinberg DA. Functional magnetic resonance imaging. Application to degenerative brain disease and hydrocephalus. Neuroimaging Clin North Am. 1995; 5: 125–134.

Barkovich AJ, Edwards MS. Applications of neuroimaging in hydrocephalus. Pediatr Neurosurg. 1992; 18: 65–83.

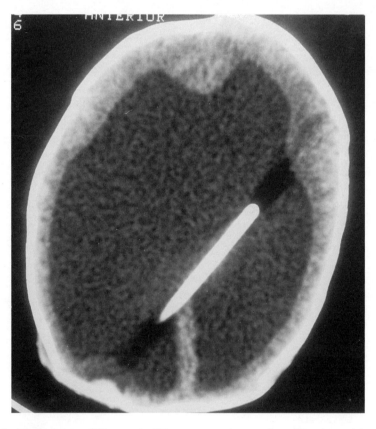

Figure 1–18 Hydrocephalus. A CT scan reveals massive dilatation of both lateral ventricles. An intraventricular shunt is present.

1.13 INCREASED INTRACRANIAL PRESSURE

Small changes in cerebral volume can usually be accommodated with little change in intracranial pressure because of the distensibility of the basilar cisterns, ventricles, and dural sinuses. After the capacity of these fluid-filled systems is reached, a small increase in intracranial volume may result in a large increase in intracranial pressure.

CT and MRI are excellent modalities to examine for evidence of increased intracranial pressure. Findings include a decrease in the size of the ventricles, a decrease or obliteration of the basal cisterns, a decrease in the size and number of cortical sulci, and herniation of brain parenchyma. Causes of increased intracranial pressure (ICP) include trauma, space-occupying lesions, hemorrhage, stroke, infection, and hydro-

cephalus. Once suspected, ICP is a neurosurgical emergency, requiring prompt ventriculostomy insertion.

SELECTED REFERENCES

Wilberger JE Jr. Outcomes analysis: intracranial pressure monitoring. Clin Neurosurg. 1997; 44: 439–448.

Golding EM, Robertson CS, Bryan RM Jr. The consequences of traumatic brain injury on cerebral blood flow and autoregulation: a review. Clin Exp Hypertens. 1999; 21: 299–332.

Stocchetti N, Rossi S, Buzzi F, et al. Intracranial hypertension in head injury: management and results. Intensive Care Med. 1999; 25: 371–376.

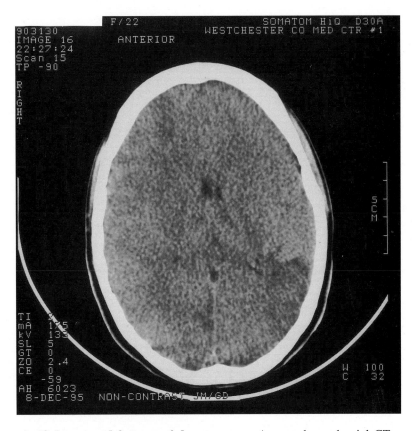

Figure 1–19 Increased intracranial pressure. A nonenhanced axial CT scan of a 22-year-old patient with anoxic brain injury shows compression of the lateral ventricles and generalized effacement of the cortical sulci. A low-density left parieto-occipital lobe infarct is also noted.

CHAPTER 2

HEAD AND NECK IMAGING

John H. Rundback, MD

Maurice R. Poplausky, MD

Bok Y. Lee, MD, FACS

2.1 NORMALS

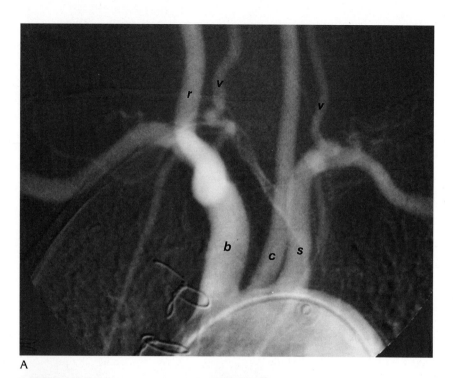

A

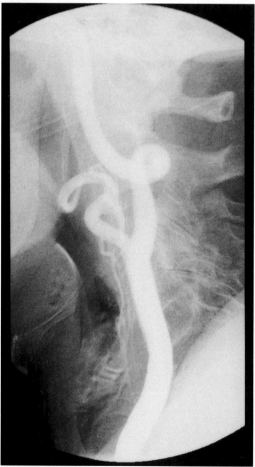

B

Figure 2–1A–C Normal carotid arteriogram. Arteriography of the thoracic aortic arch (**A**) shows the origins of the brachiocephalic (**b**), left carotid (**c**), and subclavian (**s**) arteries. The proximal portions of the right common carotid artery (**r**) and both vertebral arteries (**v**) are visualized. A selective common carotid arteriogram (**B**) shows the normal branching pattern of the carotid bifurcation and cervical segments of the internal and external carotid arteries. A coronal diagram of the anterior aspect of the neck (**C**) shows the normal relationship of the cervical vascular structures.

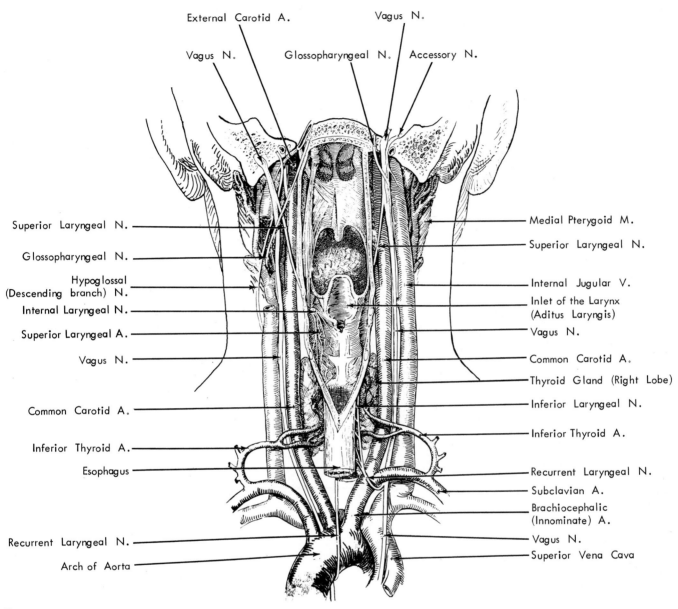

External Carotid A.

Vagus N.

Vagus N.

Glossopharyngeal N.

Accessory N.

Superior Laryngeal N.

Glossopharyngeal N.

Hypoglossal (Descending branch) N.

Internal Laryngeal N.

Superior Laryngeal A.

Vagus N.

Common Carotid A.

Inferior Thyroid A.

Esophagus

Recurrent Laryngeal N.

Arch of Aorta

Medial Pterygoid M.

Superior Laryngeal N.

Internal Jugular V.

Inlet of the Larynx (Aditus Laryngis)

Vagus N.

Common Carotid A.

Thyroid Gland (Right Lobe)

Inferior Laryngeal N.

Inferior Thyroid A.

Recurrent Laryngeal N.

Subclavian A.

Brachiocephalic (Innominate) A.

Vagus N.

Superior Vena Cava

C

2.2 ATHEROSCLEROTIC CAROTID ARTERY DISEASE

Stroke is the second leading cause of cardiovascular morbidity and mortality in the United States, accounting for approximately 700,000 cases per year, and stroke prevention and treatment represents a major health care challenge. The cause of most cerebrovascular events is embolization of debris arising from an atherosclerotic stenosis at the bifurcation of the common carotid artery and within the proximal portion of the cervical internal carotid artery. The initial screening test for carotid artery stenosis in asymptomatic patients is duplex sonography, which has a sensitivity and specificity >90% for detecting a hemodynamically significant stenosis in most series. Ultrasound findings include luminal narrowing on gray-scale images and increased spectral velocities (>120 cm/sec in the internal carotid artery) with an elevated ICA:CCA ratio on duplex interrogation. Magnetic resonance angiography (MRA) is often the initial study performed in symptomatic patients who are receiving a simultaneous magnetic resonance imaging (MRI) evaluation for intracranial disease. MRA is also useful to confirm the severity of stenosis in patients who have an abnormal ultrasound screening result, although there is a tendency for MRA to overestimate lesion severity. On MRA, a significant stenosis appears as a decreased arterial diameter and is associated with signal reduction or loss caused by turbulent flow. Neither MRI nor duplex sonography shows disease of the arch vessels or the pattern of cerebral perfusion. For these reasons, most surgeons recommend contrast arteriography before carotid revascularization. Angiography allows an assessment of the aortic arch vasculature, clearly reveals the morphology, extent, and severity of the carotid stenosis, and shows the pattern of cerebral cross-filling, which may affect treatment planning. Recently, CT angiography has also proved to be an excellent tool in providing anatomic detail of carotid bifurcation disease using 3-D reconstructions that show lumen narrowing and vessel wall irregularities.

Carotid endarterectomy (CAE) has for the past decade been the standard treatment for extracranial atherosclerotic carotid artery stenosis (CAS). The North American Symptomatic Carotid Endarterectomy Trial (NASCET) and Asymptomatic Carotid Atherosclerosis Study (ACAS) have established the benefit of CAE in reducing the risk of stroke for selected patients with carotid artery stenosis exceeding 60–70%. CAE, however, may be associated with significant morbidity (up to 18% in some series) and mortality (up to 5%), and is dependent on operator experience as a critical determinant of overall outcomes. Procedure-related morbidity includes transient ischemic attacks (TIA), disabling strokes, cranial nerve injury, bradyarrhythmias, and cervical hematomas. Recurrent stenosis is seen in up to 8% of patients after CAE, usually within the first 2 years.

In recent years, stent placement (CA-ST) has been used for the treatment of carotid bifurcation disease, and stenting is accepted by most authorities as a viable treatment option in high-risk surgical patients, patients with prior neck exploration or radiation therapy, and for carotid restenoses after CAE. The major limitation of CA-ST has been major and minor strokes, presumably caused by cerebral atheroembolization and cholesterol embolization induced by catheter and guidewire manipulation at the site of the carotid plaque. Recently, however, single center large series have shown improved results, with technical success seen in 98%, restenosis in 5%, and a 30-day major stroke rate of 3.4%. Wholey and coworkers surveyed 24 centers and recently presented the cumulative experience with extracranial carotid stent placement in 2048 patients. Technical success was achieved in 98.6%, and there was a 5% overall rate of restenosis at 6 months. Perioperative mortality was 1.4%, and the total stroke rate was 4.4%, and of these, only 1.3% were described as causing a major permanent neurologic deficit. New techniques utilizing intraprocedural cerebral protection appear to reduce the risk of stroke. These results compare favorably with those described for carotid endarterectomy. Early data suggest that advanced patient age and increasing lesion severity may increase the procedural risk of CA-ST.

SELECTED REFERENCES

North American Symptomatic Carotid Endarterectomy Trial Collaborators. Beneficial effect of carotid endarterectomy in symptomatic patients with high-grade carotid stenosis. N Engl J Med. 1991; 325: 445–453.

Executive Committee for the Asymptomatic Carotid Atherosclerosis Study. Endarterectomy for asymptomatic carotid artery stenosis. JAMA. 1995; 273: 1421–1428.

Lattimer CR, Burnand KG. Recurrent carotid stenosis after carotid endarterectomy. Br J Surg. 1997; 84: 1206–1219.

Vitek J, Iyer S, Roubin G. Carotid stenting in 350 vessels: problems faced and solved. J Invas Cardiol. 1998; 10: 311–314.

Wholey MH, Wholey M, Bergeron P, et al. Current global status of carotid artery stent placement. Cathet Cardiovasc Diagn. 1998; 44: 1–6.

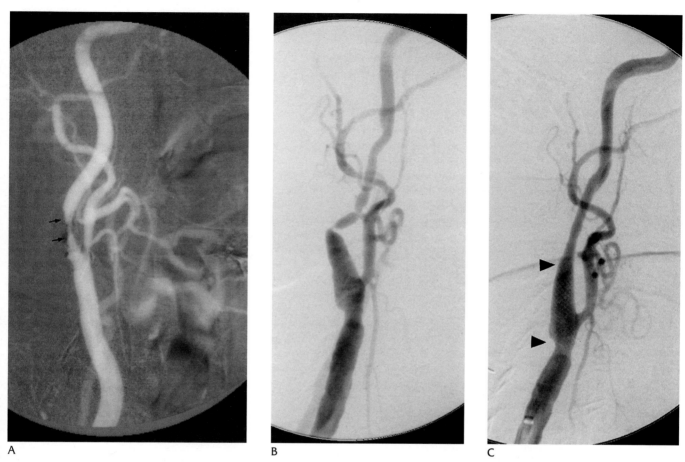

A   B   C

Figure 2–2A–C Carotid stenosis. On a selective common carotid arteriogram (**A**) of the right side, there is a severe focal concentric stenosis of the proximal internal carotid artery. Calcification within the lesion is seen adjacent to the lower arrow. A high-grade recurrent stenosis after endarterectomy in another patient (**B**) was successfully revascularized by percutaneous stent placement (**C**). The margins of the stented artery are denoted with arrowheads.

2.3 SPONTANEOUS CAROTID DISSECTION

Spontaneous dissection of the internal carotid artery (ICA) is an uncommon occurrence, although it may be responsible for up to 20% of strokes in patients younger than 45 years of age. A preponderance of these patients are women, perhaps owing to the higher incidence of fibromuscular dysplasia affecting the carotid artery in these patients. Connective tissue abnormalities are present in most cases, with the site of dissection usually beginning in the mid to upper portion of the artery. Presenting symptoms include silent ischemia, neck pain radiating to the ipsilateral jaw, cranial nerve palsies, and Horner's syndrome. The diagnosis may be made with duplex sonography, CT angiography, or magnetic resonance angiography. These modalities will reveal two vascular lumens with different patterns of flow, with compression or obstruction of antegrade flow in the true lumen commonly noted. Thrombus may be present in the false lumen, giving MRA a distinct imaging advantage because it can readily display the false lumen or intramural hematoma, suggesting the appropriate diagnosis. Angiography remains the diagnostic gold standard because it reveals tapering and obstruction of the cervical ICA extending to the petrus portion or beyond. An intimal flap is often visible, and may be severely flow-limiting.

In asymptomatic or mildly symptomatic patients with a patent ICA lumen, the usual treatment is anticoagulation. Recent published experience with endovascular stent placement suggests, however, that revascularization should be considered in these cases. For more symptomatic patients, urgent surgical or percutaneous revascularization should be performed.

SELECTED REFERENCES

Leys D, Luca C, Gobert M, et al. Cervical artery dissections. Eur Neurol. 1997; 37: 3–12.

Sidhu PS, Jonker ND, Khaw KT, et al. Spontaneous dissections of the internal carotid artery: appearances on colour doppler ultrasound. Br J Radiol. 1997; 70: 50–57.

Kirsch E, Kaim A, Engelter S, et al. MR angiography in internal carotid artery dissection: improvement of diagnosis by selective demonstration of the intramural hematoma. Neuroradiology. 1998; 40: 704–709.

Bejjani GK, Monsein LH, Laird JR, et al. Treatment of symptomatic cervical carotid dissections with endovascular stents. Neurosurgery. 1999; 44: 755–760.

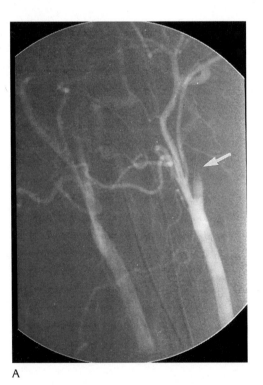
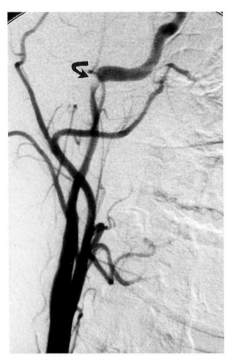

A

B

Figure 2–3A, B Carotid dissection. On a nonselective cervical arteriogram (**A**), there is a tapered occlusion of the proximal left internal carotid artery (ICA) at the lower end of the dissection flap (arrow). In contrast, a thromboembolic occlusion would appear as an abrupt cutoff resulting in a "meniscus" sign. A selective carotid arteriogram of another patient (**B**) reveals an iatrogenic dissection of the petrous portion of the ICA (curved arrow). Since the dissection did not limit antegrade flow, the patient was treated with anticoagulation only.

2.4 SUBCLAVIAN STEAL SYNDROME

Subclavian steal syndrome results from atherosclerotic stenosis or occlusion of the subclavian artery proximal to the origin of the vertebral artery. The consequent reduction in blood flow and pressure in the distal subclavian artery produces retrograde flow down the ipsilateral vertebral artery, thereby "stealing" blood from the brain stem. Although most patients are asymptomatic, characteristic symptoms relate to vertebrobasilar insufficiency (syncopal episodes, visual disturbances, ataxia) or upper extremity ischemia (differential arm pulses and blood pressures, arm pain or claudication, paresthesias, muscle wasting) that is commonly exacerbated with ipsilateral limb exercise.

In patients with suggestive symptoms, duplex ultrasonography reliably allows a diagnosis of subclavian steal syndrome to be made. Color Doppler is a valuable "localizing" step that allows identification of the vertebral artery for subsequent spectral analysis; in addition, color flow imaging facilitates determination of the direction of vertebral flow. Doppler evaluation distal to the subclavian stenosis shows dampened or monophasic axillary waveforms and retrograde flow in the vertebral artery. In cases of "partial" steal, the vertebral waveform may initially be normal or may reveal antegrade and retrograde components during the cardiac cycle (to-and-fro arterial flow). In these cases, provocative physiologic maneuvers including ipsilateral arm exercise or reactive hyperemia can create a "full" steal with corresponding Doppler abnormalities.

The initial treatment of choice in symptomatic patients is percutaneous transluminal angioplasty (PTA) with possible stent placement, which restores normal subclavian artery flow in up to 90% of patients and long-term primary patency in approximately 75%. When PTA fails or is not technically feasible, a surgical bypass (carotid-subclavian or subclavian-subclavian) can usually be performed.

SELECTED REFERENCES

Paivansalo M, Heikkila O, Tikkakoski T, et al. Duplex ultrasound in the subclavian steal syndrome. Acta Radiol. 1998; 39: 183–188.

Henry M, Amor M, Henry I, et al. Percutaneous transluminal angioplasty of the subclavian arteries. J Endovasc Surg. 1999; 6: 33–41.

Rodriguez-Lopez JA, Werner A, Martinez R, et al. Stenting for atherosclerotic occlusive disease of the subclavian artery. Ann Vasc Surg. 1999; 13: 254–260.

Sueoka BL. Percutaneous transluminal stent placement to treat subclavian steal syndrome. J Vasc Interv Radiol. 1996; 7: 351–356.

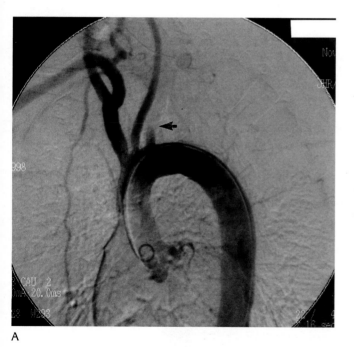
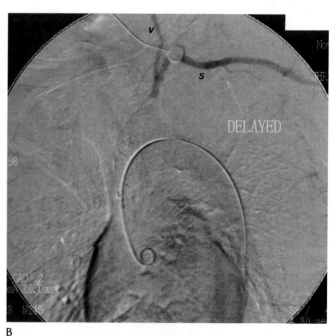

A

B

Figure 2–4A, B Subclavian steal syndrome. A thoracic aortogram (**A**) shows occlusion of the proximal left subclavian artery (short arrow). On delayed images (**B**), there is retrograde filling of the distal subclavian artery (**s**) from the left vertebral artery (**v**).

2.5 TRAUMATIC CERVICAL VASCULAR INJURY

Blunt trauma or deceleration injury to the neck may produce many vascular injuries including non–flow-limiting intimal tears, intramural hematomas, pseudoaneurysms, arteriovenous fistula formation, and arterial or venous thrombosis. Recent studies with duplex sonography suggest that these injuries may occur in up to 20% of patients sustaining severe head or cervical spine trauma, even though they are clinically asymptomatic. When arterial occlusion occurs, patients can present with symptoms of cerebral ischemia. While vascular injury in the neck can usually be diagnosed with sonography, injury to the vertebral artery at the level of the foramen transversarium is best identified using magnetic resonance imaging. In addition, MRI may be used to assess the natural history of vertebral artery lesions, although most thrombosed arteries do not spontaneously recanalize. In cases in which the diagnosis of an arterial injury is uncertain, or if surgical revascularization is contemplated, angiography will clearly show the nature and extent of any abnormality as well as the pattern of the reconstituted distal vasculature.

For penetrating injuries to the neck, the level of the injury determines how the patient is evaluated. Three cervical zones have been described: zone 1—sternal notch to the thyroid cartilage; zone 2—thyroid cartilage to the angle of the mandible, and zone 3—above the angle of the mandible to the skull base. Angiography is indicated for patients with injuries in zones 1 and 3 because of the relatively high frequency of associated vascular damage and the difficulty in clinically examining these areas adequately. Injuries to zone 2 can often be managed conservatively with careful observation and surgical exploration. In all cases, a lateral soft tissue radiograph of the neck and contrast pharyngo-esophagram (using water soluble or non-ionic contrast) should be considered to exclude the presence of associated pharyngeal or esophageal injury.

SELECTED REFERENCES

Rommel O, Niedeggen A, Tegenthoff M, et al. Carotid and vertebral artery injury following severe head or cervical spine trauma. Cerebrovasc Dis. 1999; 9: 202–209.

Weller SJ, Rossitch E Jr, Malek AM. Detection of vertebral artery injury after cervical spine trauma using magnetic resonance angiography. J Trauma. 1999; 46: 660–666.

Friedman D, Flanders A, Thomas C, Millar W. Vertebral artery injury after acute cervical spine trauma: rate of occurrence as detected by MR angiography and assessment of clinical consequences. Am J Roentgenol. 1995; 164: 443–447.

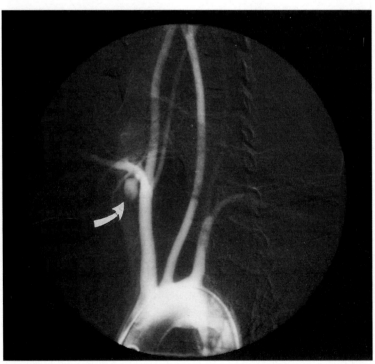

A

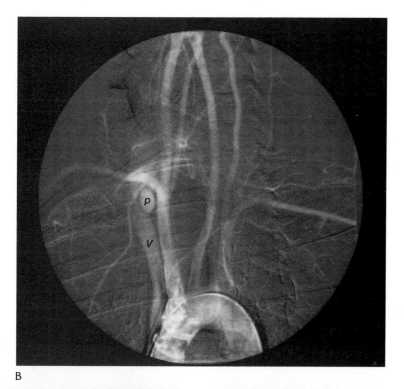

B

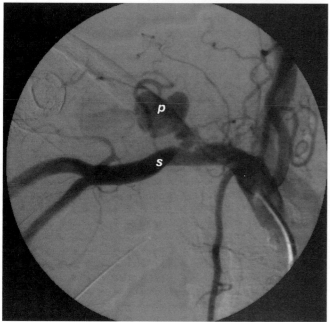

C

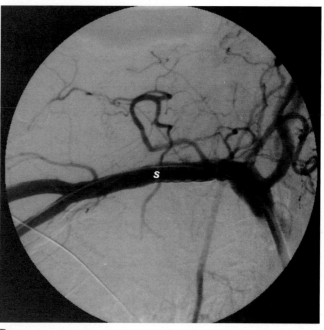

D

Figure 2–5A–D Traumatic vascular injury. Early (**A**) and late (**B**) arteriograms in a patient sustaining a stab wound to the right side of the neck. A traumatic pseudoaneurysm is noted to arise from the inferior aspect of the proximal subclavian artery (arrow). Late images reveal the pseudoaneurysm (**p**) and early opacification of the right brachiocephalic vein (**V**) due to an arteriovenous fistula. A second patient (**C**) with a subclavian artery pseudoaneurysm after a misplaced central venous catheter was successfully treated by placement of a polytetrafluoroethylene-covered stent graft (**D**). (**s** represents subclavian artery.)

2.6 APPROACH TO THE CERVICAL SPINE RADIOGRAPH

The cross-table lateral radiograph of the cervical spine is usually obtained first. If this is normal, the completion series is then performed including anterior-posterior, odontoid, and flexion-extension views when appropriate. All 7 cervical vertebrae must be visualized in their entirety for a complete study. A systematic approach for the evaluation of cervical spine radiographs is necessary.

Lateral radiograph

The prevertebral soft tissues should be evaluated first. The thickness of the prevertebral soft tissues in the upper cervical spine, as measured from the posterior aspect of the tracheal air column to the anterior vertebral body, should be less than 1 vertebral body width. An increase in this soft tissue space with a history of trauma may indicate hematoma, and should increase the suspicion of an associated cervical spine fracture. Other causes of retropharyngeal and prevertebral soft tissue swelling include abscesses and neoplasm.

Four nearly parallel smooth lines representing the normal structures of the cervical spine should be evaluated next for discontinuity. The first line, representing the anterior spinal ligament, is drawn along the anterior aspect of the vertebral bodies, and should be smooth and uninterrupted. Although disruption of this anterior spinal line may be associated with serious cervical spine injury, osteophytes due to degenerative spondylosis may also cause this finding. In these cases, cervical alignment is otherwise maintained, and there is no associated prevertebral soft tissue swelling. The second line follows the posterior aspect of the vertebral bodies and represents the posterior longitudinal ligament. The third line, called the spinolaminar line, follows the anterior aspect of the spinous processes. The spinal cord resides between the 2nd and 3rd lines, and any irregularity may thus imply the presence of bony impingement on the spinal cord. The fourth line connects the posterior aspect of the spinous processes, and represents the ligamentum nuchae and interspinous ligaments.

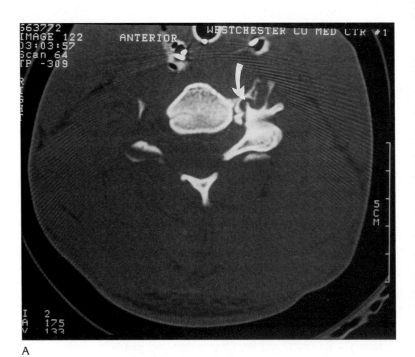

A

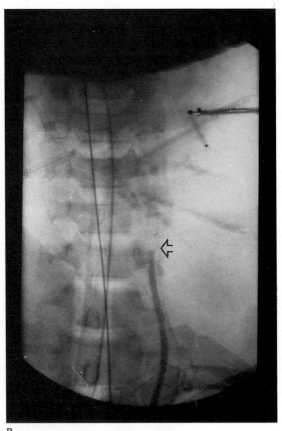

B

Figure 2–6A, B Traumatic vertebral artery injury in a patient with a cervical spine fracture. A comminuted fracture of the lateral mass of C5 is seen on an axial CT scan (**A**). A retropulsed fracture fragment extends into the left transverse foramina of C6 (arrow), which is the normal position of the vertebral artery. A selective vertebral arteriogram (**B**) of the left side shows thrombotic occlusion of the artery at the level of the injury (open arrow).

The osseous structures should then be evaluated for any fractures, which can appear as linear lucencies or as compressed or sclerotic bone.

Next, the atlantoaxial joint should be evaluated. This is done by measuring the distance between the posterior aspect of the arch and the dens. This should not measure more than 3 mm in adults (up to 5 mm in children). Measurements greater than these in the setting of trauma indicate injury to the transverse ligament. Other causes include ligamentous laxity, commonly seen in patients with rheumatoid arthritis.

Lastly, the disc spaces should be evaluated for unusually wide or narrowed spacing. It is important to keep in mind that degenerative diseases also commonly cause disc space narrowing.

Odontoid view

The dens should first be evaluated for any fractures. Next, the lateral masses should be examined to see whether they are equidistant from the dens on both sides. If not, this is indicative of an injury. In addition, the lateral masses of C1 should align with the lateral masses of C2. A fracture of C1 is present if its lateral masses "overhang" the lateral masses of C2.

Anterior-posterior view

Any irregularities or fractures not visible on the lateral radiograph will often be visible on the AP view. Two radiographs at 90° orthogonal projections should always be performed when evaluating for a fracture.

SELECTED REFERENCES

El-Khoury GY, Kathol MH, Daniel WW. Imaging of acute injuries of the cervical spine: value of plain radiography, CT and MR imaging. Am J Roentgenol. 1995; 164: 43–50.

Tehranzadeh J, Palmer S. Imaging of cervical spine trauma. Semin Ultrasound CT MR. 1996; 17: 93–104.

Kathol MH. Cervical spine trauma. What is new? Radiol Clin North Am. 1997; 35: 507–532.

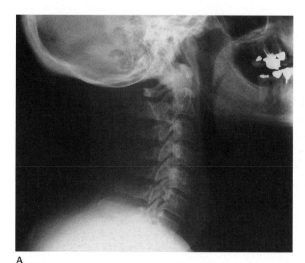

A

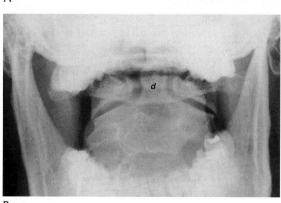

B

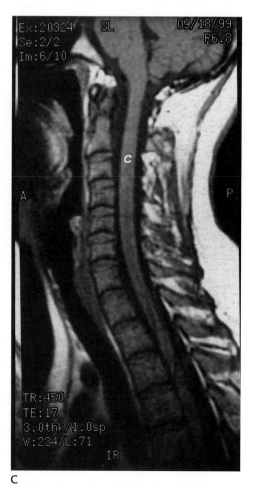

C

Figure 2–7A–C Normal cervical spine. The normal alignment of the vertebral bodies is noted on lateral (**A**) and odontoid view (**B, d** represents dens) radiographs of the cervical spine. A midsagittal MRI (**C**) shows the spinal cord (**c**) and paraspinal ligaments.

2.6.1 Jefferson Burst Fracture

The classic Jefferson burst fracture consists of four fractures: two fractures involving the anterior arch of C1, and two fractures involving the posterior arch of C1. Jefferson burst fractures are caused by an axial force that is transmitted from the occipital condyles of the skull to the lateral masses of C1, splitting them apart. Since C1 is a bony ring, it breaks in multiple places. This injury is considered stable unless there is associated disruption of the transverse ligament. Neurologic injury occurs infrequently.

Jefferson burst fractures are best detected on the open mouth odontoid projection. The lateral masses of C1 are seen overhanging the margins of the C2 body bilaterally. When the sum of the overhang of each lateral mass is >9 mm, the transverse ligament is also ruptured. CT is excellent for revealing fractures of the atlas and should be performed when the plain film diagnosis is uncertain.

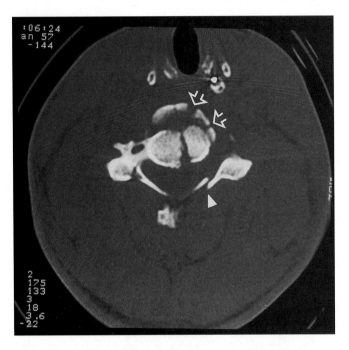

Figure 2–8 Jefferson burst fracture. An axial cervical CT scan of the axis (C2) shows multiple comminuted displaced fractures in the vertebral body (open arrows) and posterior elements (arrowhead).

2.6.2 Atlantoaxial Dissociation

Atlanto-occipital dislocation is almost always immediately fatal. It is the result of a severe shear injury that causes separation of the cranium from the spine. In almost all cases, the skull is anteriorly displaced relative to the cervical vertebrae. Death usually results from transection of the medulla caused by compression between the opisthion of the skull base and the odontoid process. Surviving patients uniformly have severe permanent neurologic damage and associated soft tissue injury.

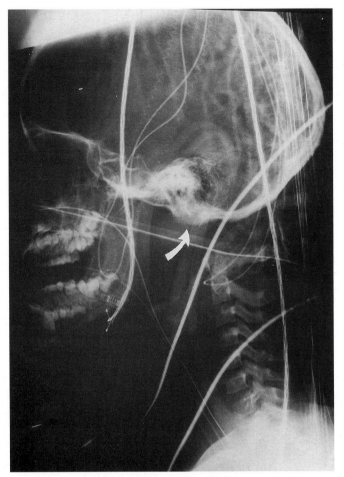

Figure 2–9 Atlantoaxial dissociation. On a lateral radiograph of the cervical spine, there is separation and displacement of the articular masses of the skull base (curved arrow) relative to the C1 vertebral body.

2.6.3 Hangman's Fracture

A hangman's fracture is an unstable fracture of the posterior elements of C2 (the axis) with anterior displacement of C2 on C3. The mechanism of injury involves an abrupt hyperextension of the neck. As the name implies, these fractures can result from hanging, although they more commonly occur today as a result of a motor vehicle accident (hitting one's head on the dashboard). Hangman's fractures account for about 7% of all cervical injuries. Patients who sustain this type of injury usually escape neurologic impairment because the fracture of the posterior elements "decompresses" the injured area. Simultaneous hyperflexion injuries of the lower cervical spine are common, and maybe due to "rebound" hyperflexion occurring at the time of injury.

This type of injury is best diagnosed with the lateral plain radiograph. Varying degrees of anterior spondylolisthesis of C2 on C3 is shown along with diastasis, kyphosis, and retropharyngeal swelling. CT is helpful in those patients with neurologic compromise and reveals fractures of the posterior ring of C2. Coronal or 3-D reconstructions will also reveal the loss of normal alignment of C2 on C3.

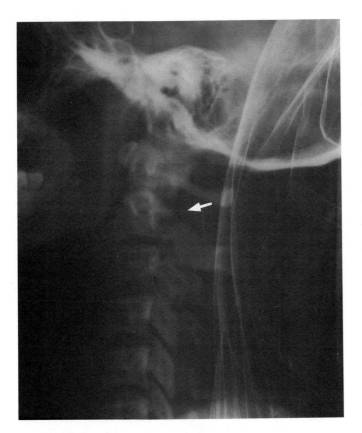

Figure 2–10 Hangman's fracture. A lateral view of the
~~cervical spine shows lucency extending~~ across the posterior
~~arch of C2 in an~~ attempted hanging.

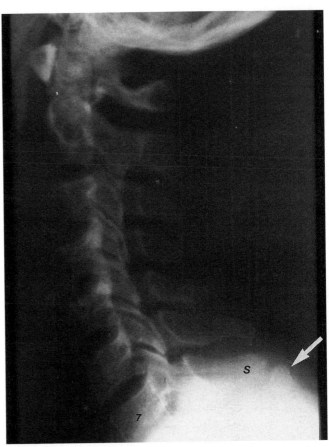

Figure 2–11 Clay-shoveler's fracture. A lateral film of the
neck shows a displaced osseous fragment (arrow) due to a
fracture of the C7 spinous process (**S**).

2.6.5 Facet Dislocation

Facet dislocation, also referred to as a "locked facet," characteristically occurs with simultaneous hyperflexion and rotation,
and accounts for approximately 4% of all cervical spine injuries. The cervical spine between the C4 and C7 levels is most
commonly involved; unilateral facet dislocation occurs more
commonly than bilateral dislocations. The injury results in rupture of the ligaments of the apophyseal joints articulating adjacent vertebral bodies, and the superior pillar slides forward
over the inferior pillar to ultimately rest in the intervertebral
foramen. The interspinous ligament is always ruptured. When
in the "locked position," this injury is considered stable. Once
reduced, the spine is usually unstable and requires fixation for
healing.

Multiple radiographic views, including oblique projections,
are necessary to define this entity. The oblique projection best
displays the dislocated facet while the anteroposterior projection shows the rotational component of this injury (visualized
as rotation of the spinous processes below the level of injury).
The involved disc space is usually widened with the inferior
vertebral body posteriorly located in relation to the superior
vertebral body. CT displays the relationship of the facets, making the diagnosis apparent.

he spinous process of
a clay-shoveler's frac-
ere is a strong associ-
hyperflexion sprains.
ominantly at the base
on and the pull of the
nterspinous ligament.
secondary to the at-
e name for this type of
rkers who would toss
ulders; the clay would
great force on the lig-
of the spine and even-

is the most helpful for
letely corticated bone
s processes. A fracture
be seen. Focal hyper-
mild spondylolisthesis
nces may indicate the
sprain.

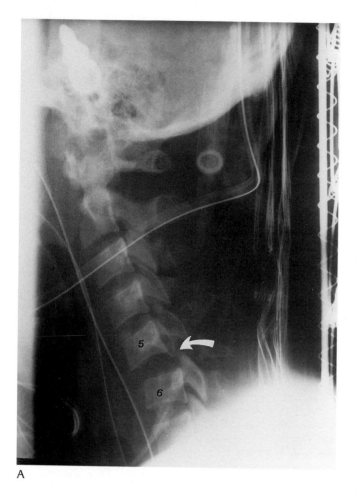

A

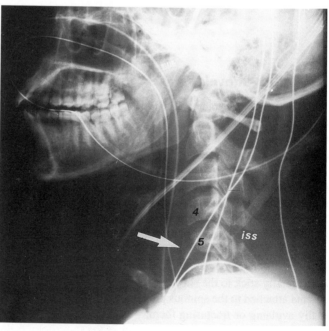

B

Figure 2–12A, B Facet dislocation. Anterior dislocation of the inferior facet of C5 relative to C6 (**A**, curved arrow) results in disruption of the normal cervical lines, hyperflexion, and separation of the posterior elements at the level of the injury. A sagittally reconstructed CT image (**B**) clearly depicts the inferior C5 facet to be positioned within the neural foramen on the left side (arrow). Further images showed bilateral facet dislocation.

2.6.6 Flexion Teardrop

A flexion teardrop fracture can occur after a severe forced flexion of the cervical spine, for example, as a result of motor vehicle accidents or from diving into shallow water. The forced flexion disrupts the posterior ligaments and causes a compression fracture of the anterior portion of the vertebral body. The fractured fragment is characteristically triangular in shape and arises from the anterior inferior surface of the vertebral body. Posterior displacement of the upper spine may also be seen because of posterior longitudinal ligament disruption. Flexion teardrop fractures are considered unstable, and are commonly associated with spinal cord injury from a retropulsed fragment of the posterior portion of the vertebral body impinging on the spinal canal and cord.

Flexion teardrop fractures can be easily recognized on the standard lateral radiograph of a cervical spine series. Anterior wedging of the vertebral body with an associated fracture of the anterior inferior vertebral body is seen. As in all cases where the presence of a cervical spine injury is in question on the cervical spine series, a CT scan through the area in question with reconstructed images is invaluable.

Figure 2–13 Flexion teardrop fracture. A lateral radiograph of the cervical spine reveals cortical compression and an anteriorly displaced marginal fracture (arrow) of the C5 vertebral body. Widening of the C4 through C5 interspinous space (**iss**) due to disruption of the posterior longitudinal ligament is also noted.

2.7 SPINAL CORD INJURY

Injury to the spinal cord can occur without disruption of the osseous structures, although spondylosis (with degenerative osteophytes) is often present. Injuries such as spinal cord contusions and nerve root avulsions cannot be diagnosed with plain film radiography or routine CT scanning, but are usually revealed with MRI, myelography, or CT myelography.

MRI best displays the edema associated with spinal cord contusions; the edema appears as central low-signal intensity lesions on T_1-weighted images and increased signal on T_2-weighted images. Hemorrhage can be seen as low signal on gradient echo images. Myelography or CT myelography will show swelling of the cord and resultant displacement of contrast filling the subdural space, but will not directly visualize the cord injury. Syringomyelia can occur as a late complication of spinal contusions and will appear as a central low-attenuation lesion on CT or as a cystic, fluid-filled space on MRI.

Nerve root avulsions can occur with injuries to the upper extremities and pelvis, with distraction forces severing or stretching the nerve roots at their origins from the cord. The dural sleeve is usually injured as well, forming a pseudomeningocele. MRI may actually display the avulsed nerve root with an adjacent fluid-filled structure representing the pseudomeningocele. CT myelography shows the pseudomeningocele as contrast extending outside the dura matter of the spinal canal and partially filling the dural nerve sac.

When bony spine injuries are present, the primary goal is to identify mechanical cord compression caused by bone fragments, disc herniation, spinal stenosis and epidural hematomas, so that surgical decompression can be rapidly performed. MRI is the preferred imaging modality for identifying these kinds of associated injuries.

SELECTED REFERENCES

Rao SC, Fehlings MG. The optimal radiologic method for assessing spinal canal compromise and cord compression in patients with cervical spinal cord injury. Part I: an evidence-based analysis of published literature. Spine. 1999; 24: 598–604.

Fehlings MG, Rao SC, Tator CH, et al. The optimal radiologic method for assessing spinal canal compromise and cord compression in patients with cervical spinal cord injury. Part II: results of a multicenter study. Spine. 1999; 24: 605–613.

Selden NR, Quint DJ, Patel N, et al. Emergency magnetic resonance imaging of cervical spinal cord injuries: clinical correlation and prognosis. Neurosurgery. 1999; 44: 785–792.

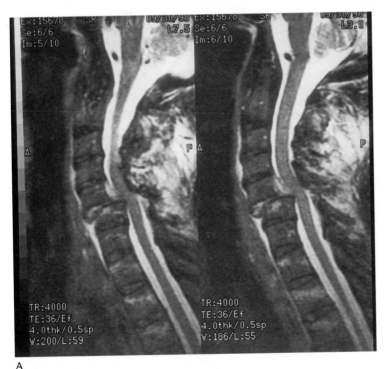

A

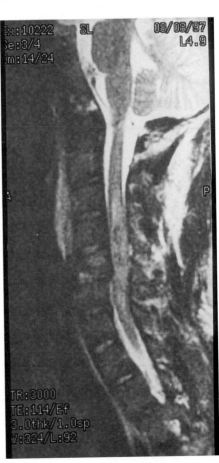

B

Figure 2–14A, B Spinal-cord injury. A midsagittal T_1-weighted cervical MRI shows a fracture dislocation of C5 through C6. Retrolisthesis of the C6 vertebral body causes compression and deformity of the cervical cord. A T_2-weighted image of another patient (**B**) reveals a heterogeneous pattern and areas of increased signal within the cord at the site of a cervical injury. These findings represent early edema due to neural damage.

CHAPTER 3

CHEST IMAGING

Maurice R. Poplausky, MD

John H. Rundback, MD

Bok Y. Lee, MD, FACS

3.1 NORMALS

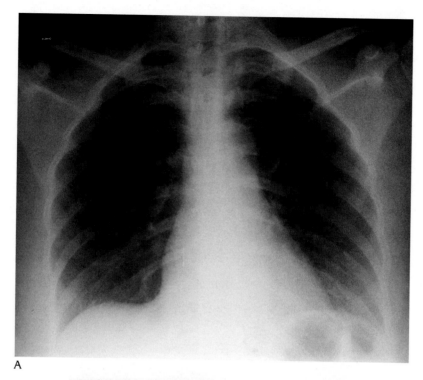

A

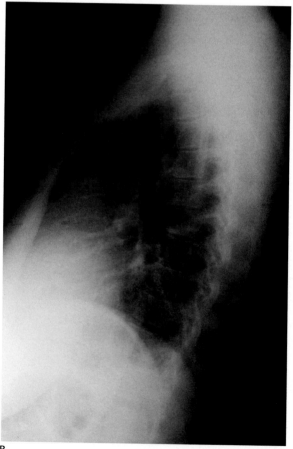

B

Figure 3–1A, B Posteroanterior and lateral radiographs of the normal chest.

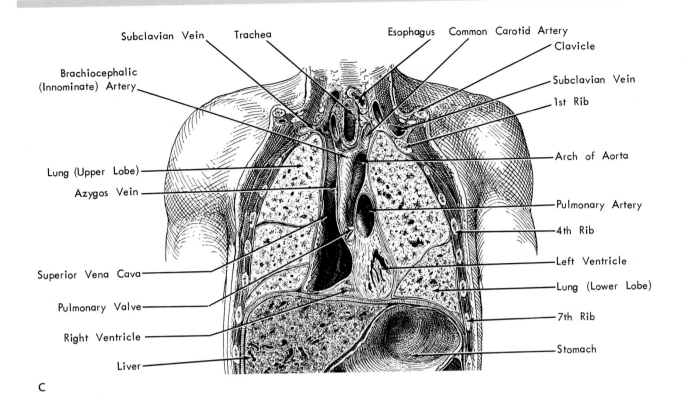

C

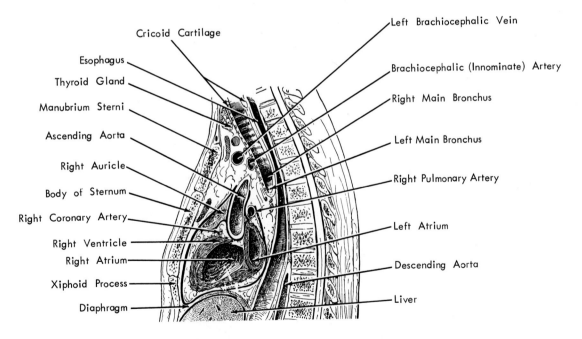

D

Figure 3–1C, D Corresponding sectional drawings show normal anatomic structures and lobar anatomy of the lung.

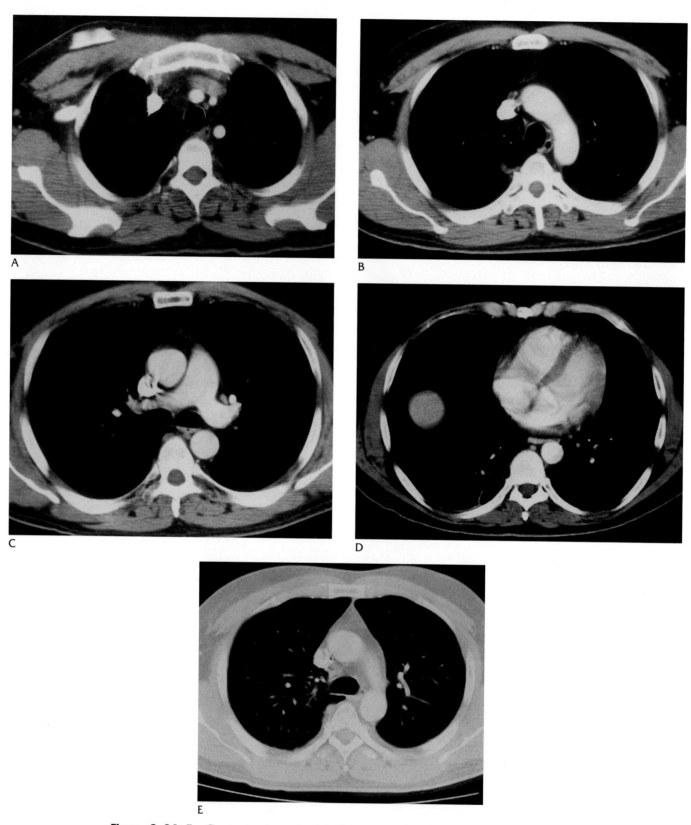

Figure 3–2A–E Contrast-enhanced axial CT scans at the level of the great vessels (**A**), see opposite page; aortic arch (**B**), see page 46; pulmonary artery (**C**), see page 47; and heart (**D**), see page 48. Normal pulmonary vascular markings are well delineated using different window and level settings (**E**).

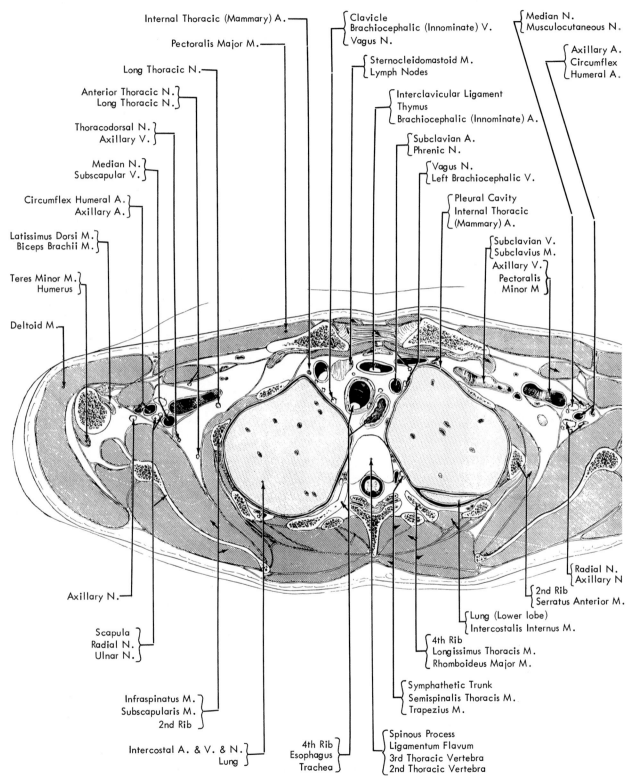

Internal Thoracic (Mammary) A.

Pectoralis Major M.

Long Thoracic N.

Anterior Thoracic N.
Long Thoracic N.

Thoracodorsal N.
Axillary V.

Median N.
Subscapular V.

Circumflex Humeral A.
Axillary A.

Latissimus Dorsi M.
Biceps Brachii M.

Teres Minor M.
Humerus

Deltoid M.

Clavicle
Brachiocephalic (Innominate) V.
Vagus N.

Sternocleidomastoid M.
Lymph Nodes

Interclavicular Ligament
Thymus
Brachiocephalic (Innominate) A.

Subclavian A.
Phrenic N.

Vagus N.
Left Brachiocephalic V.

Pleural Cavity
Internal Thoracic
(Mammary) A.

Median N.
Musculocutaneous N.

Axillary A.
Circumflex
Humeral A.

Subclavian V.
Subclavius M.
Axillary V.
Pectoralis
Minor M

Radial N.
Axillary N

2nd Rib
Serratus Anterior M.

Lung (Lower lobe)
Intercostalis Internus M.

4th Rib
Longissimus Thoracis M.
Rhomboideus Major M.

Symphathetic Trunk
Semispinalis Thoracis M.
Trapezius M.

Spinous Process
Ligamentum Flavum
3rd Thoracic Vertebra
2nd Thoracic Vertebra

Axillary N.

Scapula
Radial N.
Ulnar N.

Infraspinatus M.
Subscapularis M.
2nd Rib

Intercostal A. & V. & N.
Lung

4th Rib
Esophagus
Trachea

F

Figure 3–2F–I Anatomic drawings, corresponding to Figures 3–2A–D, show normal correlative anatomy.

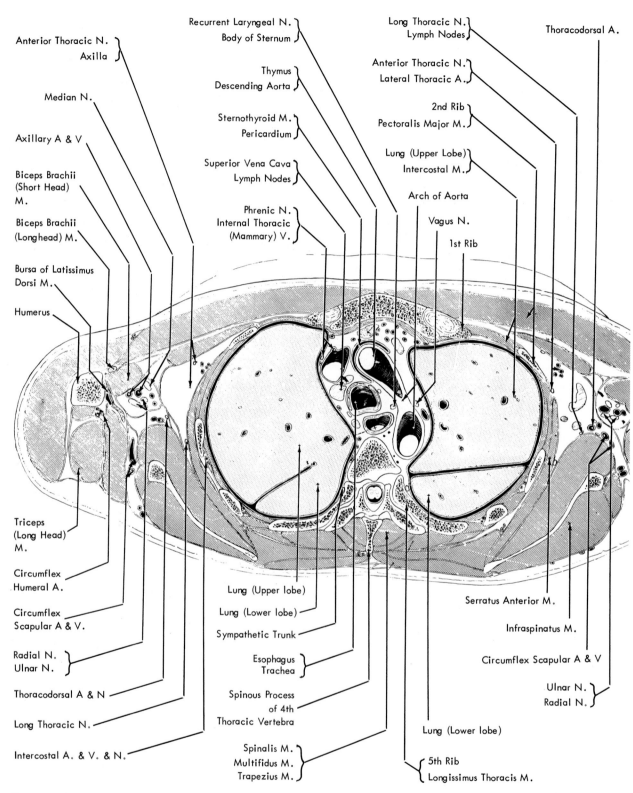

Anterior Thoracic N.
Axilla

Median N.

Axillary A & V

Biceps Brachii
(Short Head)
M.

Biceps Brachii
(Longhead) M.

Bursa of Latissimus
Dorsi M.

Humerus

Triceps
(Long Head)
M.

Circumflex
Humeral A.

Circumflex
Scapular A & V.

Radial N.
Ulnar N.

Thoracodorsal A & N

Long Thoracic N.

Intercostal A. & V. & N.

Recurrent Laryngeal N.
Body of Sternum

Thymus
Descending Aorta

Sternothyroid M.
Pericardium

Superior Vena Cava
Lymph Nodes

Phrenic N.
Internal Thoracic
(Mammary) V.

Lung (Upper lobe)

Lung (Lower lobe)

Sympathetic Trunk

Esophagus
Trachea

Spinous Process
of 4th
Thoracic Vertebra

Spinalis M.
Multifidus M.
Trapezius M.

Long Thoracic N.
Lymph Nodes

Anterior Thoracic N.
Lateral Thoracic A.

2nd Rib
Pectoralis Major M.

Lung (Upper Lobe)
Intercostal M.

Arch of Aorta

Vagus N.

1st Rib

Thoracodorsal A.

Serratus Anterior M.

Infraspinatus M.

Circumflex Scapular A & V

Ulnar N.
Radial N.

Lung (Lower lobe)

5th Rib
Longissimus Thoracis M.

G

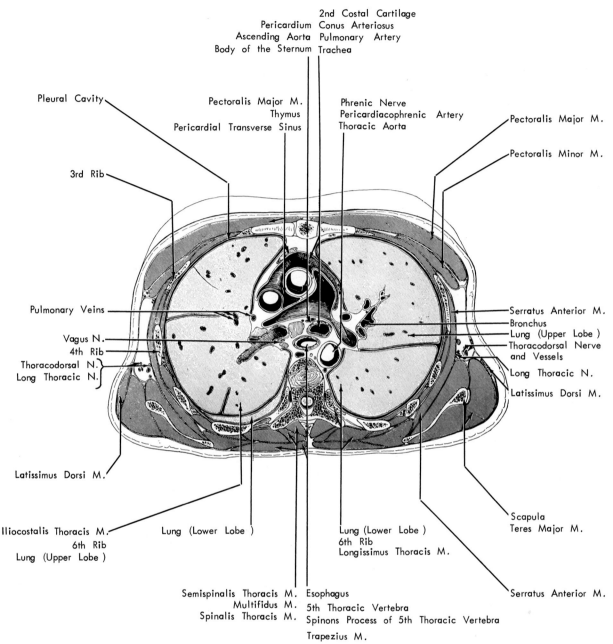

2nd Costal Cartilage
Pericardium Conus Arteriosus
Ascending Aorta Pulmonary Artery
Body of the Sternum Trachea

Pleural Cavity

Pectoralis Major M.
Thymus
Pericardial Transverse Sinus

Phrenic Nerve
Pericardiacophrenic Artery
Thoracic Aorta

Pectoralis Major M.

Pectoralis Minor M.

3rd Rib

Pulmonary Veins

Serratus Anterior M.
Bronchus
Lung (Upper Lobe)
Thoracodorsal Nerve
and Vessels
Long Thoracic N.
Latissimus Dorsi M.

Vagus N.
4th Rib
Thoracodorsal N.
Long Thoracic N.

Latissimus Dorsi M.

Scapula
Teres Major M.

Iliocostalis Thoracis M.
6th Rib
Lung (Upper Lobe)

Lung (Lower Lobe)

Lung (Lower Lobe)
6th Rib
Longissimus Thoracis M.

Serratus Anterior M.

Semispinalis Thoracis M.   Esophagus
Multifidus M.   5th Thoracic Vertebra
Spinalis Thoracis M.   Spinons Process of 5th Thoracic Vertebra

Trapezius M.

H

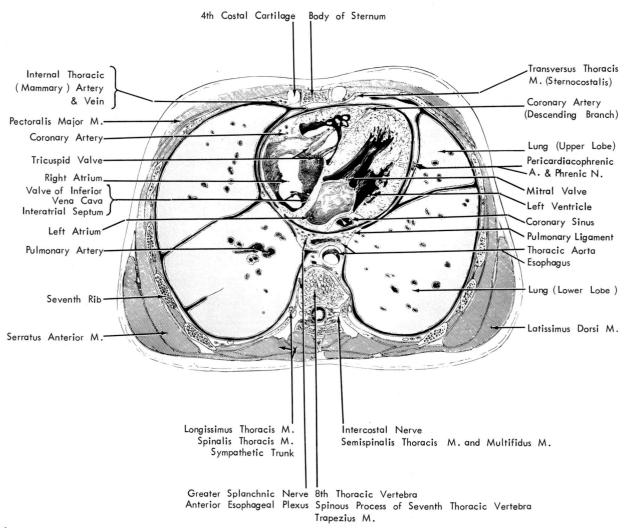

4th Costal Cartilage   Body of Sternum

Internal Thoracic
(Mammary) Artery
& Vein

Pectoralis Major M.

Coronary Artery

Tricuspid Valve

Right Atrium

Valve of Inferior
Vena Cava
Interatrial Septum

Left Atrium

Pulmonary Artery

Seventh Rib

Serratus Anterior M.

Transversus Thoracis
M. (Sternocostalis)

Coronary Artery
(Descending Branch)

Lung (Upper Lobe)

Pericardiacophrenic
A. & Phrenic N.

Mitral Valve

Left Ventricle

Coronary Sinus

Pulmonary Ligament

Thoracic Aorta

Esophagus

Lung (Lower Lobe)

Latissimus Dorsi M.

Longissimus Thoracis M.
Spinalis Thoracis M.
Sympathetic Trunk

Intercostal Nerve
Semispinalis Thoracis M. and Multifidus M.

Greater Splanchnic Nerve   8th Thoracic Vertebra
Anterior Esophageal Plexus   Spinous Process of Seventh Thoracic Vertebra
Trapezius M.

I

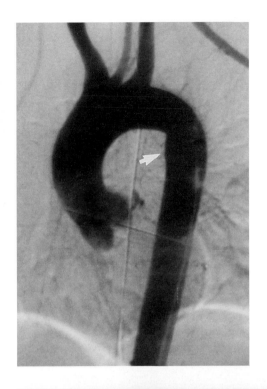

Figure 3–3 Normal thoracic aortogram obtained in the left anterior oblique projection. The origins of the great vessels are clearly seen. Note the slight prominence of the proximal descending aorta caused by the normal ductus bump (arrow).

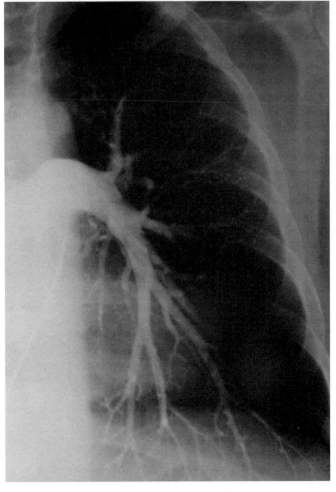

Figure 3–4 Normal selective pulmonary arteriogram of the left lung.

3.2 AORTIC RUPTURE

Traumatic aortic tears are uncommon injuries, but when they do occur, the associated morbidity and mortality are very high. Proposed mechanisms of injury include shearing caused by the sudden deceleration of the mobile and fixed portions of the aorta and compression of the aorta between the sternum and spine. This kind of injury is usually associated with motor vehicle accidents. While traumatic aortic tears often occur at the aortic root, these patients usually die before arriving at the hospital. In most patients the tear is located at the aortic isthmus, just distal to the left subclavian artery origin and proximal to the ligamentum arteriosus. Traumatic tears also occur in the descending aorta at the level of the diaphragm, but these are much less common. Although the term "aortic transection" has been used, only 40% of injuries are transmural (extending through all three layers of the aortic wall).

The workup for a traumatic aortic injury begins with a good chest radiograph. A normal mediastinum virtually eliminates the possibility of an aortic tear (with a negative predictive value of >97%). A widened mediastinum (>8 cm in diameter) is a sensitive (although not specific) radiographic sign of acute aortic injury. Other loosely associated signs include tracheal deviation, nasogastric tube deviation, first rib fractures, and a left apical cap. If a widened mediastinal is found, the patient should proceed to spiral CT. Positive findings include mediastinal hematoma and pseudoaneurysm formation. If an aortic tear cannot be ruled out by the spiral CT, a thermic aortogram should be performed. Positive angiographic findings include wall irregularity, intimal flaps, pseudoaneurysm formation, and delayed emptying. Extravasation of contrast is a rare finding.

SELECTED REFERENCES

Duhaylongsod FG, Glower DD, Wolfe WG. Acute traumatic aortic aneurysm: the Duke experience from 1970 to 1990. J Vasc Surg. 1992; 15: 331–342.

Stark P, Jacobson F. Radiology of thoracic trauma. Curr Opin Radiol. 1992; 4: 87–93.

Creasy JD, Chiles C, Routh WD, Dyer RB. Overview of traumatic injury of the thoracic aorta. Radiographics. 1997; 17: 27–45.

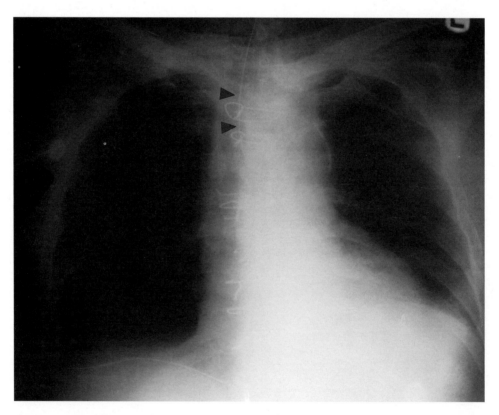

Figure 3–5 Aortic rupture. A portable chest radiograph shows slight widening of the mediastinum and deviation of the nasogastric tube toward the right side (arrowheads). Note the sternal wires from previous sternotomy.

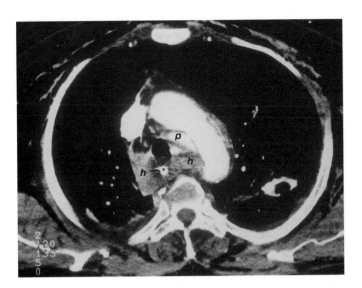

Figure 3–6 Aortic rupture. A contrast-enhanced CT image at the level of the aortic arch shows a pseudoaneurysm (**p**) as an extraluminal contrast collection contiguous with the aorta. A mediastinal hematoma is also present (**h**). A nasogastric tube and left chest tube are noted.

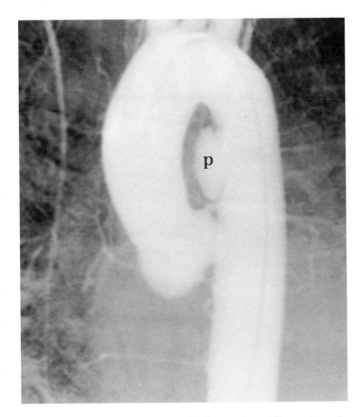

Figure 3–7 Aortic rupture. Left anterior oblique thoracic aortogram shows disruption of the intima and a pseudoaneurysm (**p**) at the aortic isthmus.

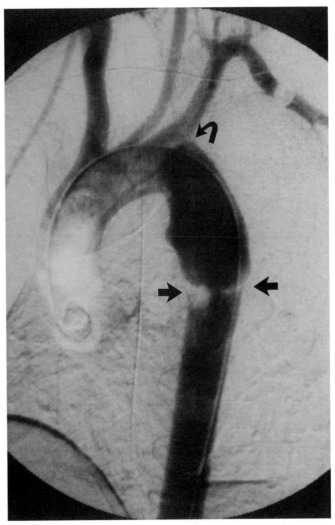

Figure 3–8 Aortic rupture. A thoracic aortogram of another patient shows a complete transection of the proximal descending thoracic aorta (arrows). There is retrograde extension to the origin of the subclavian artery (curved arrow).

3.3 AORTIC DISSECTION

Spontaneous dissection of the aorta typically begins in the thoracic aorta, and may extend caudally to involve the abdominal aorta. Stanford type A dissections involve the ascending aorta or aortic arch and require emergent surgical repair. In contrast, type B dissections arise distal to the origin of the left subclavian artery, and are medically managed by controlling coexistent hypertension. Radiographs of the chest may show mediastinal widening, pleural effusions, indistinctness of the aortic arch, or displacement of intimal calcifications; however, plain films may be normal in as many as 25% of cases. Computed tomography (CT), CT angiography, and conventional or digital subtraction angiography demonstration of an intimal flap separating the true and false lumens is the sine qua non of aortic dissection. Collapse of the true lumen caused by loss of elastin content and relatively sluggish flow within the false lumen may also be seen. In addition, angiography may show com-

plications including aortic insufficiency, extension into the abdominal aorta, branch vessel occlusion, and visceral ischemia that would require more definitive management. The recent development of percutaneous septal fenestration and the introduction of intravascular stents may in selected cases restore perfusion to obstructed visceral branches and allow minimally invasive therapy for ischemic complications.

SELECTED REFERENCES

Svensson LG, Labib SB. Aortic dissection and aortic aneurysm surgery. Curr Opin Cardiol. 1994; 9: 191–199.

Sanders C. Current role of conventional and digital aortography in the diagnosis of aortic disease. J Thorac Imaging. 1990; 5: 48–59.

Williams DM, Lee DY, Hamilton BH, et al. The dissected aorta: percutaneous treatment of ischemic complications—principles and results. J Vasc Interv Radiol 1997; 8: 605–625.

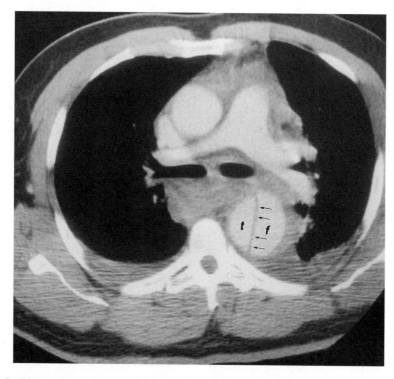

Figure 3–9 Type B aortic dissection. Contrast-enhanced CT image at the level of the main pulmonary artery. An intimal flap (arrows) within the descending thoracic aorta separates the larger false lumen (**f**, laterally) and smaller true lumen (**t**, medially). Visualization of an intimal flap is the hallmark of an aortic dissection.

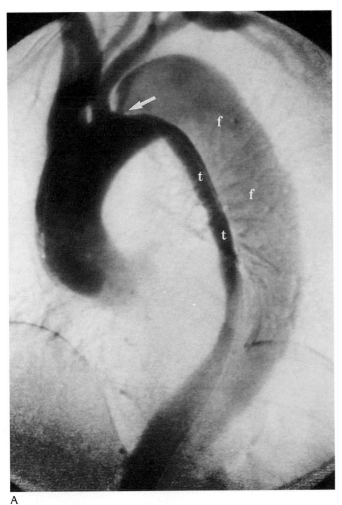

A

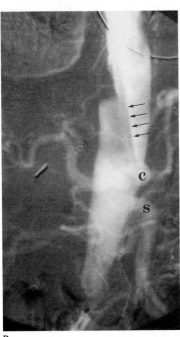

B

Figure 3–10A, B Type B aortic dissection. Thoracic (**A**) and abdominal (**B**) aortograms. In the thoracic aortogram, the contrast enters the false lumen (**f**) just distal to the subclavian artery. The site of intimal disruption is marked with an arrow. The catheter is within the collapsed true lumen (**t**). In the abdominal aortogram of another patient, a dissection flap (small arrows) is seen extending to the celiac axis (**c** represents celiac axis; **s**, superior mesenteric artery).

Figure 3–11 Aortic dissection. Sagittal MRA. A long dissection flap is easily recognized (arrowheads). MRI has the advantage of providing images of the aorta in multiple planes.

3.4 THORACIC AORTIC ANEURYSM

Aortic aneurysms may involve the thoracic or abdominal aorta, and occur as a result of atherosclerosis, vasculitis (eg, Takayasu's), or a connective tissue disease (eg, Marfan's syndrome, cystic medial necrosis, homocystinuria, Ehlers-Danlos syndrome). "True" aneurysms of the aorta result from degeneration and thinning of all three layers of the aortic wall, and may be fusiform (circumferential) or saccular (eccentric) in nature. For thoracic aortic aneurysms, the imaging appearance and location of the aneurysm (as well as clinical information) may be suggestive of the underlying cause: atherosclerotic—irregularity of the remainder of the aorta and its major branches; Marfan's syndrome, cystic medial necrosis—dilatation of the

sinotubular junction, aortic insufficiency; syphilis—ascending aorta, "tree bark" appearance; and Takayasu's arteritis—occlusion or stenosis of the aortic arch branch vessels.

Complications of thoracic aneurysms are dissection, transient ischemic attacks or strokes, rupture, and symptoms resulting from local mass effect.

SELECTED REFERENCES

Pitt MP, Bonser RS. The natural history of thoracic aortic aneurysm disease: an overview. J Card Surg. 1997; 12 (suppl 2): 270–278.

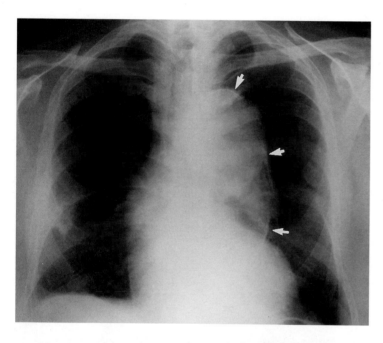

Figure 3–12 Thoracic aortic aneurysm. A chest radiograph reveals a chronic aneurysm of the arch and descending thoracic aorta. Calcification in the aortic wall is clearly evident (arrows).

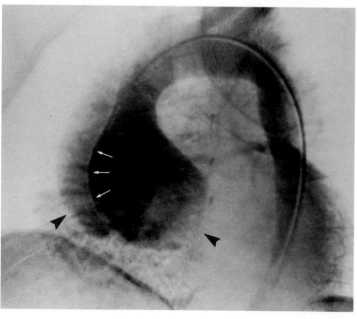

Figure 3–13 Thoracic aortic aneurysm. Aortogram of a patient with Marfan's syndrome showing dilatation of the aortic sinuses (arrowheads) and proximal ascending aorta with an associated type A dissection (arrows). Involvement of the aortic sinuses distinguishes Marfan's from other causes of type A dissection.

3.5 INFECTIOUS (MYCOTIC) AORTIC ANEURYSM

Infectious or mycotic aneurysms occur when intima injured as a result of atherosclerosis, trauma, surgery, or iatrogenic causes is exposed to and colonized by bacteria either by the contiguous spread of infection or by embolic seeding from a remote source. The bacteria eventually weakens the aortic wall, resulting in aneurysm formation. Risk factors include intravenous drug abuse, immune compromise, and bacterial endocarditis. Commonly implicated organisms are staphylococcal, streptococcal, and enterococcal species.

Mycotic aneurysms can be either true or false aneurysms. They are usually eccentric and saccular and are commonly located in the ascending aorta. They are commonly multiple and involve the aorta and/or its major branch vessels (renal arteries, superior mesenteric artery, iliac arteries). There is a high tendency to rupture. On CT, MRI, and ultrasound, mycotic aneurysms appear as a focal vascular dilation or a contiguous extraluminal contrast collection. The saccular shape, location (branch point), multiplicity, and clinical history all help to make the correct diagnosis. Angiography is used to confirm the presence of an aneurysm and its relationship to branch vessels.

SELECTED REFERENCES

Walsh DW, Ho VB, Haggerty MF. Mycotic aneurysm of the aorta: MRI and MRA features. J Magn Reson Imaging. 1997; 7: 312–315.

Wilde CC, Tan L, Cheong FW. Computed tomography and ultrasound diagnosis of mycotic aneurysm of the abdominal aorta due to Salmonella. Clin Radiol. 1987; 38: 325–326.

Pasic M. Mycotic aneurysm of the aorta: evolving surgical concept. Ann Thorac Surg. 1996; 61: 1053–1054.

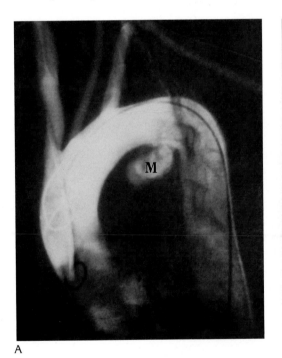
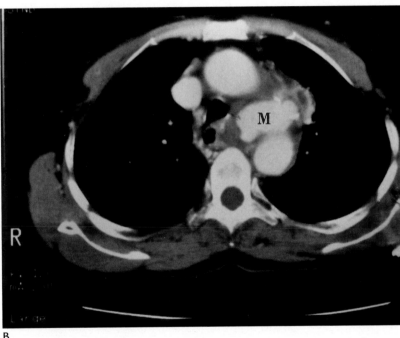

A   B

Figure 3–14A, B Mycotic pseudoaneurysm. A thoracic aortogram (**A**) and CT scan (**B**) show an irregular collection of contrast inferior to the aortic arch caused by a mycotic pseudoaneurysm (**M**). The aorta above and below the pseudoaneurysm appears normal.

3.6 PENETRATING ATHEROSCLEROTIC ULCER

A penetrating atherosclerotic ulcer (PAU) is a distinct clinico-pathologic entity that most commonly affects the descending thoracic aorta. Patients with this condition present with pain radiating to the back or symptoms of peripheral thromboembolism. PAUs may also serve as an entry site for spontaneous aortic dissection with the resultant risk of ischemic symptoms due to branch vessel occlusion. The diagnosis is made by cross-sectional imaging or angiography, which demonstrates a focal projection of contrast from the lateral aspect of the aortic wall.

The natural untreated history of PAU is aneurysmal degeneration of the affected aortic segment.

SELECTED REFERENCES

Movsowitz HD, Lampert C, Jacobs LE, Kotler MN. Penetrating atherosclerotic aortic ulcers. Am Heart J. 1994; 128: 1210–1217.

Coady MA, Rizzo JA, Hammond GL, et al. Penetrating ulcer of the thoracic aorta: What is it? How do we recognize it? How do we manage it? J Vasc Surg. 1998; 27: 1006–1016.

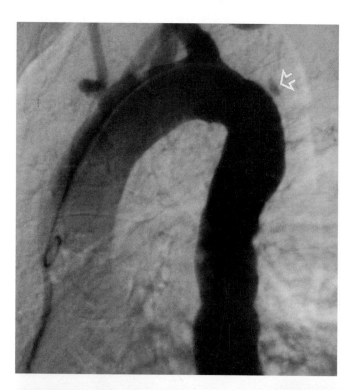

Figure 3–15 Penetrating atherosclerotic ulcer. Oblique thoracic aortogram shows a focal "button-like" projection of contrast (open arrow) just lateral to the distal arch. There is moderate atherosclerosis of the remainder of the aorta.

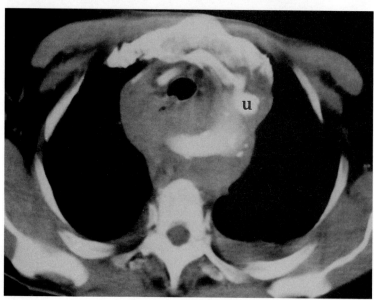

Figure 3–16 Penetrating atherosclerotic ulcer. A CT of the same patient shows the ulcer (**u**) to communicate with the aortic arch. A large mediastinal hematoma is seen.

3.7 AORTIC COARCTATION

Coarctation of the aorta is a congenital narrowing of the aorta. It can involve any portion of the aorta, but most commonly involves the aortic arch. It can also vary in severity from a slight stenosis to atresia. Aortic coarctation is divided into the more common postductal or adult type and a preductal or infantile type. With the postductal type, the stricture is focal and located at or just beyond the ligamentum arteriosus. With the preductal type, the stricture is usually longer and extends from just distal to the brachiocephalic artery to the level of the ductus arteriosus. This type is often associated with other congenital cardiovascular anomalies.

Aortic coarctation can be diagnosed by many different radiographic modalities including chest radiographs, ultrasound, MRI, and angiography. Plain film findings include rib notching, the "high" aortic knob sign, and the "3" sign. Rib notching, representing erosion of the inferior aspect of the ribs, is caused by dilated intercostal arteries that reconstitute flow to the aorta distal to the coarctation. The "3" sign is caused by an indentation in the normally smooth contour of the descending thoracic aorta.

The relationship of the aortic stricture to the great vessels can be evaluated easily and safely using MRI, and any associated anomalies can be simultaneously evaluated. T_1 sagittal images are generally the most useful images. The role of angiography to detect aortic coarctation in patients has changed significantly with the emergence of MRI. Angiography may be used to show anatomic detail not seen on MRI and to obtain pressure gradients across the lesion to assess the hemodynamic severity. Percutaneous intervention with balloon angioplasty has been performed successfully in many institutions, but has yet to gain widespread acceptance.

SELECTED REFERENCES

Rao PS. Coarctation of the aorta. Semin Nephrol. 1995; 15: 87–105.

Rao PS, Chopra PS. Role of balloon angioplasty in the treatment of aortic coarctation. Ann Thorac Surg. 1991; 52: 621–631.

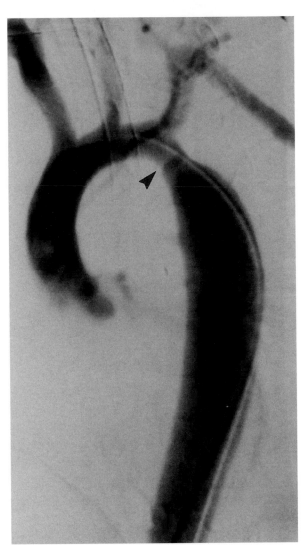

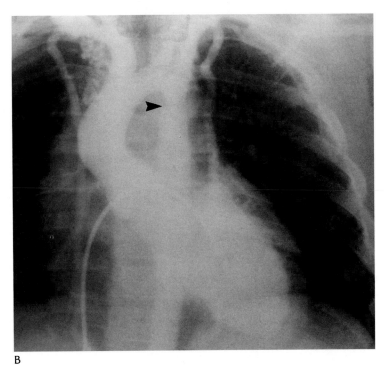

B

Figure 3–17A, B Adult type aortic coarctation. Aortograms of two different patients reveal focal narrowing of the aorta near the ligamentum arteriosus (arrowheads). Note the presence of ventricular hypertrophy and prominent arterial collaterals in **B**.

A

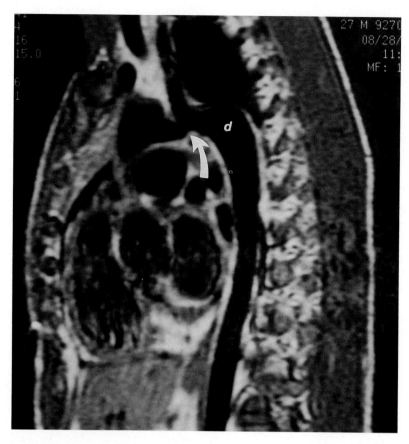

Figure 3–18 Aortic coarctation. A sagittal MRI shows an atypical coarctation of the aortic arch proximal to the subclavian artery (curved arrow). There is poststenotic dilatation of the proximal descending thoracic aorta (**d**).

3.8 HEMOPTYSIS

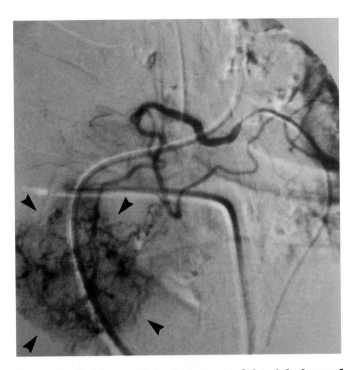

Figure 3–19 A bronchial arteriogram of the right lung of a patient with massive hemoptysis due to bronchogenic lung carcinoma. A hypervascular lung mass is seen (arrowheads) which was subsequently successfully embolized.

Although alarming to both patient and physician, most acute episodes of hemoptysis cease spontaneously and are moderate in volume. Massive hemoptysis is defined as bleeding exceeding 600 mL/24 h, and should be considered a life-threatening emergency. In the United States, cystic fibrosis is the most common cause of hemoptysis in children and young adults, whereas tumors are the most common cause in the elderly. Infections such as tuberculosis are the most common cause worldwide. Bronchiectasis is a less frequent cause.

The bronchial arteries are the most common source of bleeding in a patient with hemoptysis; a pulmonary artery source is responsible in approximately 10% of cases. Bronchography or high resolution CT scanning is often helpful in localizing the site of the bleeding before angiography is performed. Selective arteriography of the bronchial arteries is the gold standard for excluding or defining the source and cause of bleeding. Findings include arterial enlargement (>3 mm), arteriopulmonary shunting, active contrast extravasation, tumor neovascularity, and abnormally tortuous vessels. If a bleeding site is identified, transcatheter embolization should be performed, with care taken to avoid occluding spinal arterial branches. Bleeding can be successfully controlled after embolotherapy in 80% of cases.

SELECTED REFERENCES

Cahill BC, Ingbar DH. Massive hemoptysis. Assessment and management. Clin Chest Med. 1994; 15: 147–167.

Thompson AB, Teschler H, Rennard SI. Pathogenesis, evaluation, and therapy for massive hemoptysis. Clin Chest Med. 1992; 13: 69–82.

Roberts AC. Bronchial artery embolization therapy. J Thorac Imaging. 1990; 5: 60–72.

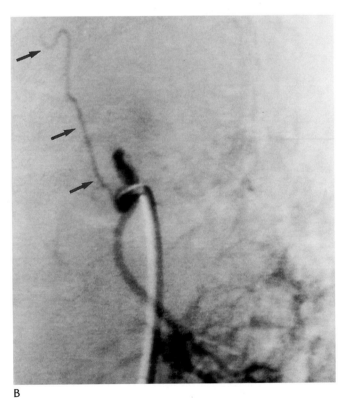

B

Figure 3–20A, B Bronchial artery embolization. Bronchial arteriography of a patient with hemoptysis shows enlargement and tortuosity of the bronchial artery and parenchymal hypervascularity (**A**). After partial transcatheter embolization, an anterior spinal artery with its characteristic hairpin loop is now apparent (**B**, arrows). No further embolization was attempted.

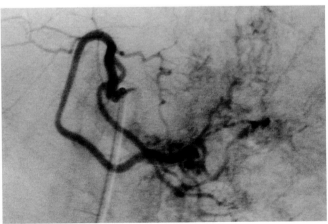

A

3.9 PULMONARY PSEUDOANEURYSM SECONDARY TO SWAN–GANZ CATHETER

Pulmonary pseudoaneurysms are rare causes of hemoptysis most commonly caused by penetrating trauma to the lung. An increasing number of iatrogenic pulmonary pseudoaneurysms following the insertion of a Swan–Ganz catheter have been recently described. The presumed cause is inflation of the balloon on a catheter that has been inadvertently wedged into a branch of the pulmonary artery, resulting in arterial rupture. Patients with a Swan–Ganz catheter in place who present with hemoptysis should have an emergent pulmonary angiogram performed. A saccular collection of contrast is seen at the site of rupture. Contrast can occasionally be identified entering the bronchial tree. When a pseudoaneurysm is found, the treatment of choice is embolization of the pseudoaneurysm.

SELECTED REFERENCES

Ferretti GR, Thony F, Link KM, et al. False aneurysm of the pulmonary artery induced by a Swan–Ganz catheter: clinical presentation and radiologic management. AJR. 1996; 167: 941–945.

Ray CE, Kaufman JA, Geller SC, et al. Embolization of pulmonary catheter-induced pulmonary artery pseudoaneurysms. Chest. 1996; 110: 1370–1373.

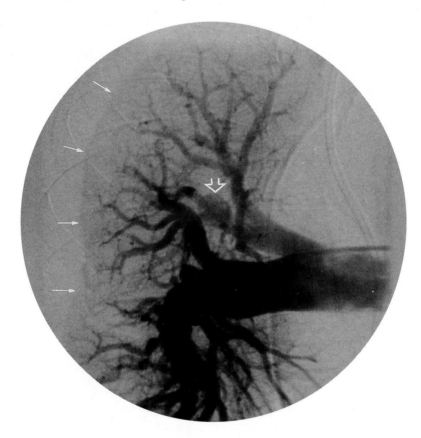

Figure 3–21 Swan–Ganz catheter-induced pulmonary pseudoaneurysm. A selective pulmonary arteriogram of the right lung reveals a well-circumscribed pseudoaneurysm (open arrow) at the site of balloon inflation in a branch of the right middle lobe pulmonary artery. Displacement of the opacified lung margin by a pleural effusion is incidentally noted (small arrows).

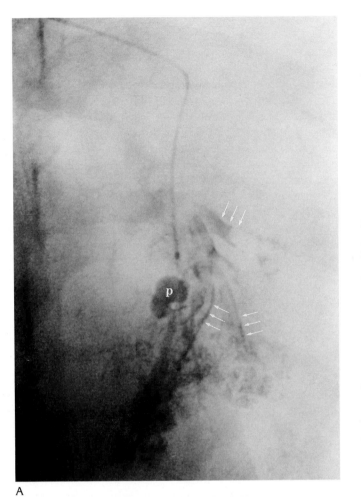

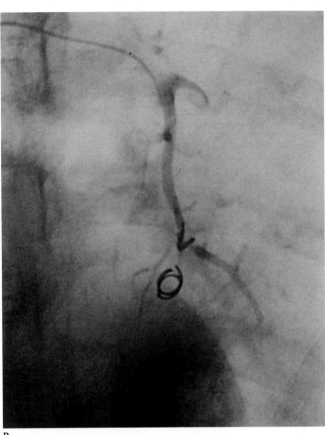

A

B

Figure 3–22A, B Swan–Ganz catheter-induced pulmonary pseudoaneurysm.
Superselective lower lobe pulmonary angiography (**A**) shows a pseudoaneurysm (**p**) and
contrast staining of the bronchial tree (arrows). After coil embolization (**B**), the pseudoaneurysm and bronchi are no longer visible.

3.10 ACUTE PULMONARY EMBOLISM

Pulmonary embolism (PE) is a highly prevalent and often underdiagnosed condition, accounting for approximately 25% of in-hospital deaths. PE occurs as a complication of deep venous thrombosis (DVT), usually of the lower extremities, although venous duplex imaging of patients with known PE is normal in 50% of cases. Emboli are often multiple and bilateral, and have a predilection for the lower lobes. In patients without underlying pulmonary compromise, approximately 25% of the lung volume needs to be affected for symptoms to develop. Death occurs if 60% or more of the pulmonary vascular bed is acutely obstructed. Symptoms and signs include chest pain (pleurisy), dyspnea, tachypnea, hypoxemia, hypocapnia, hemoptysis, an elevated arterial-alveolar gradient, and electrocardiographic abnormalities. Radiographs of the chest frequently demonstrate nonspecific abnormalities, including diaphragmatic elevation, small pleural effusions, or small areas of linear atelectasis or consolidation. Focal oligemia (Westermark's sign) or a pleural-based density reflecting a pulmonary infarct (Hampton's hump) are occasionally seen.

The diagnosis of acute PE may be confirmed by ventilation-perfusion lung scanning or spiral CT. However, in cases of indeterminate or intermediate probability scans, or when there is a discrepancy between imaging findings and the clinical suspicion of acute PE, angiography remains the gold standard for diagnosis. While pulmonary angiography is generally safe and easily performed, extra care must be exercised with patients who have elevated right ventricular pressures, significant pulmonary hypertension, or ventricular irritability. Patients with a left bundle branch block will need to have a temporary pacemaker placed before the procedure. The hallmark of acute PE on angiography is an intraluminal filling defect or abrupt vessel cutoff. Other signs are pulmonary hypertension, focal arterial spasm, segmental oligemia, and segmental absence of venous drainage from the affected portion of the lung.

Treatment for acute PE is systemic anticoagulation. When anticoagulation is contraindicated or breakthrough PE occurs, an inferior vena cava filter is effective in preventing recurrent emboli. Percutaneous fluoroscopic-guided aspiration thromboembolectomy, systemic (intravenous) and catheter-directed thrombolytic therapy, and surgical thrombectomy are reserved for instances of life-threatening PE, and may allow more rapid restoration of pulmonary arterial flow and improved oxygen saturation in selected patients. However, the long-term benefits of these procedures in terms of improved pulmonary function and increased patient survival is not yet determined.

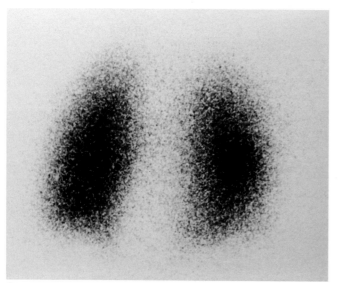

A

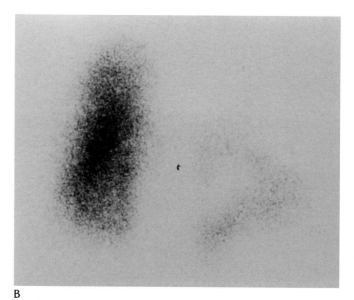

B

Figure 3–23A, B Acute pulmonary embolism. Ventilation/perfusion (V/Q) lung scan. A posterior scintiscan of the lungs (**A**) obtained after the inhalation of Kr 89 gas shows nearly normal ventilation. Corresponding perfusion images using Tc 99m-labeled microaggregated albumin particles (**B**) show a large mismatch and multiple segmental areas of diminished and absent perfusion in the middle and upper lobes of the right lung.

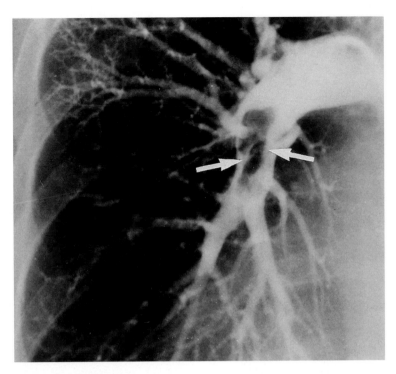

Figure 3–24 Acute pulmonary embolism. A selective pulmonary arteriogram of the right lung reveals a large intraluminal filling defect within the interlobar pulmonary artery (arrows). This filling defect causes a "tram track" appearance and abrupt vessel cutoff of the lateral basal and middle lobe arteries.

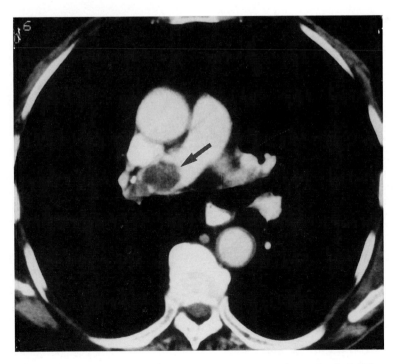

Figure 3–25 Acute pulmonary embolism. A contrast-enhanced spiral CT scan at the level of the pulmonary artery on the right lung shows a large intravascular filling defect (arrow) consistent with an acute embolus.

3.11 CHRONIC PULMONARY EMBOLISM

Chronic pulmonary embolism is a sequela of recurrent acute PE, and therefore occurs more frequently in patients at risk for DVT. Patients with chronic PE have a continuously deteriorating clinical course complicated by pulmonary hypertension and congestive heart failure, resulting in eventual death. Treatment is aimed at correcting hypercoagulability or other comorbid medical conditions predisposing to DVT. Diagnostic tests are of limited value and are generally used to evaluate for a suspected new episode of PE. Radiographs of the chest may show diffuse parenchymal abnormalities and prominence of the central pulmonary vessels with an abrupt change in caliber more peripherally ("pruned tree appearance"). Angiography will allow plethysmographic measurements of pulmonary hypertension (PA pressures >40 mm Hg), and will show prominent central vessels, tortuous peripheral vasculature, multiple irregular arterial webs, strictures and stenoses, and a pattern of focal oligemia with segmental absence of venous drainage.

SELECTED REFERENCES

Handler JA, Reied CF. Acute pulmonary embolism. Aggressive therapy with anticoagulants and thrombolytics. Postgrad Med. 1995; 97: 61–62, 65–68, 71–72.

Greenspan RH. Pulmonary angiography and the diagnosis of pulmonary embolism. Prog Cardiovasc Dis. 1994; 37: 93–105.

Worsley DF, Alavi A. Comprehensive analysis of the results of the PIOPED study. Prospective Investigation of Pulmonary Embolism Diagnosis Study. J Nucl Med. 1995; 36: 2380–2387.

Cotroneo AR, Di Stasi C, Cina A. Interventional radiology in the treatment of pulmonary embolism. Rays (Milano). 1996; 21: 417–424.

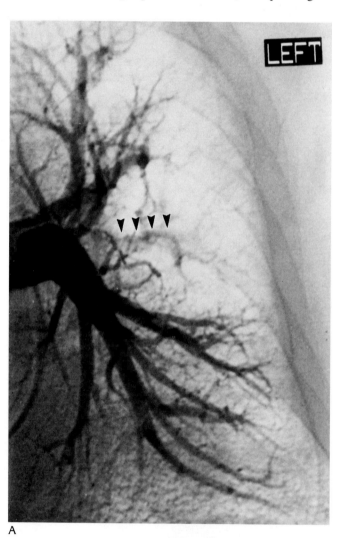

A

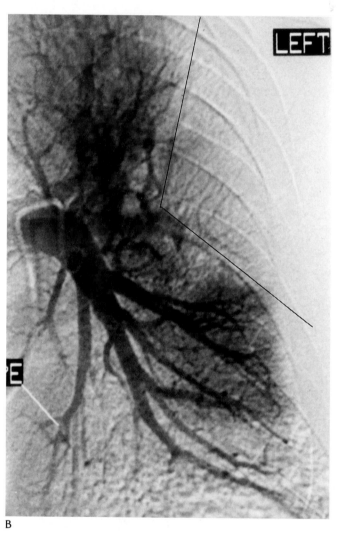

B

Figure 3–26A, B Chronic pulmonary embolism. Early and late arterial images from a pulmonary arteriogram of the left lung show partial recanalization of the lingular artery (**A**, arrowheads) and an associated focal wedge-shaped area of parenchymal oligemia (**B**, lines).

3.12 EMPYEMA

An empyema is a postinfectious inflammatory disease of the pleura resulting in an accumulation of pus in the pleural space. Pulmonary infections are the most common cause of empyema, and anaerobic bacteria are the most frequent microorganisms found. Postpneumonic empyemas usually occur along the posterior pleural space or within a fissure. In the acute stage, there is an inflammatory process occurring in the adjacent lung. In more chronic stages, the adjacent lung may appear normal and the empyema is more clearly defined. Air within an empyema may indicate a bronchopleural fistula, a pleurocutaneous fistula, or an infection with a gas-producing organism.

Radiography of the chest and CT are the best radiologic modalities to help identify an empyema. On chest radiographs, acute empyemas cannot be distinguished from simple pleural effusions. Layering of fluid is seen, which has obtuse margins with the chest wall. Blunting of the costophrenic angle can also be seen if the empyema is not loculated. With chronic empyemas, a thick pleural peel can be seen, which may become calcified. A contrast-enhanced CT is helpful in differentiating between a lung abscess and an empyema. On CT, an empyema is usually oval or lenticular as compared with a lung abscess, which is usually round. The wall enhances with contrast and is usually smooth, well defined, and of uniform thickness. The wall of an abscess is usually irregular and of variable thickness. Parietal and visceral pleural separation, called the "split pleura" sign, can also be seen with empyemas.

The only diagnostic tool to definitively confirm that the pleural fluid represents an empyema is thoracentesis. Since the fluid collections are usually loculated, ultrasound guidance may be necessary for successful fluid aspiration.

SELECTED REFERENCES

Cowens ME, Johnston MR. Thoracic empyema: causes, diagnosis, and treatment. Compr Ther. 1990; 16: 40–45.

Lee RB. Radiologic evaluation and intervention for empyema thoracis. Chest Surg Clin North Am. 1996; 6: 439–460.

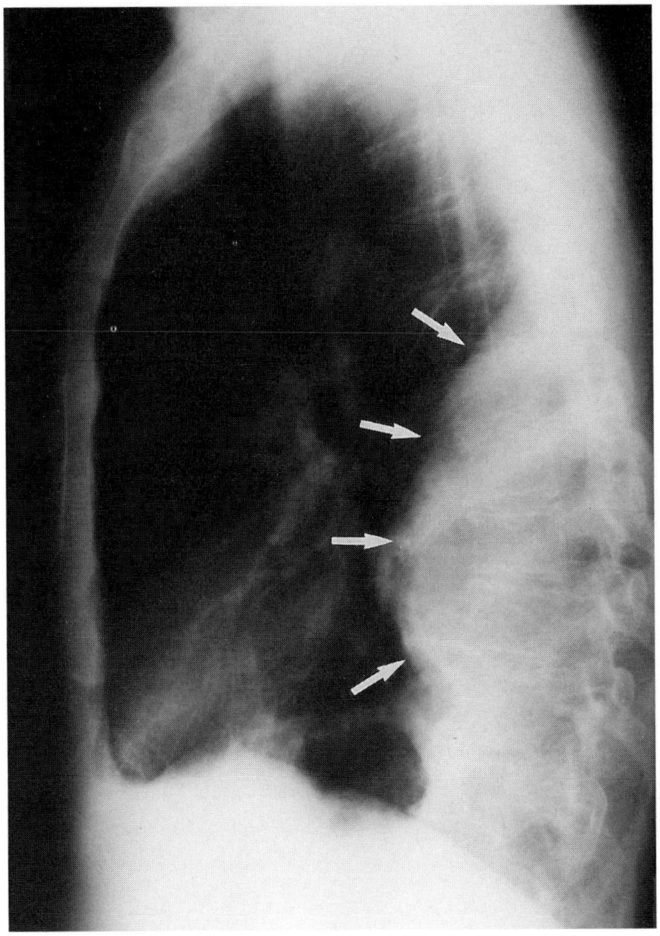

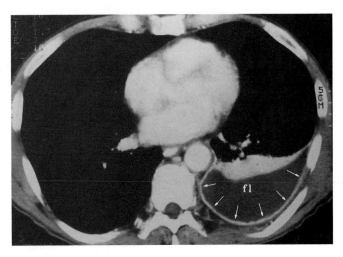

Figure 3–28 Empyema. A chest CT scan in the same patient shows a posterior fluid collection (**fl**) causing passive atelectasis of the adjacent left lung. Enhancement of the pleura (small arrows) surrounding the fluid is indicative of an empyema rather than a simple pleural effusion.

Figure 3–27 Empyema. A lateral chest film shows a loculated convex extrapleural density overlying the dorsal spine (arrows).

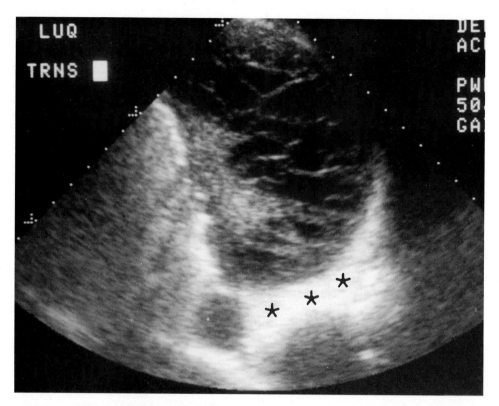

Figure 3–29 Empyema.   Ultrasound reveals a multiseptated, complex cystic mass within the pleural space consistent with an empyema. Enhanced through-transmission, seen as increased echogenicity deep to the mass (asterisks), confirms the cystic nature of the lesion.

3.13 LUNG ABSCESS

Lung abscesses represent necrotic cavities in the pulmonary parenchyma occurring as a result of necrotizing pneumonia (gram-negative and *Staphylococcus aureus*), anaerobic lung infections (eg, aspiration), septic emboli, cavitating lung tumors, or tuberculosis. The appropriate diagnosis is determined by the clinical setting, sputum cultures, blood cultures, and radiographs or computed tomographic scans of the chest. Bronchoscopy may be necessary for patients with an unusual presentation or for those who fail to respond to therapy. Antibiotics are the mainstay of treatment, although drainage of the abscess cavity may be required for resistant infections. Complications of lung abscesses include hemoptysis, development of a bronchopulmonary fistula, empyema formation, and secondary fungal superinfection.

Chest radiography and CT are the modalities of choice when evaluating pulmonary abscesses. Radiographic findings include a solitary mass (if the abscess is completely fluid filled), a cavity with an air-fluid level, or a cavitary infiltrate. A pyogenic abscess must be differentiated from cavitary tuberculosis or a cavitating carcinoma. Early CT scans may show a central area of low attenuation representing necrosis within the lung parenchyma. Well-developed abscesses on CT are poorly defined, spherically shaped lesions with irregularly thick walls. A distinct finding in abscess cavities is that pulmonary vessels course through the mass rather than being displaced.

SELECTED REFERENCES

Wiedemann HP, Rice TW. Lung abscess and empyema. Semin Thorac Cardiovasc Surg. 1995; 7: 119–128.

Klein JS, Schultz S, Heffner JE. Interventional radiology of the chest: image-guided percutaneous drainage of pleural effusions, lung abscess, and pneumothorax. AJR. 1995; 164: 581–588.

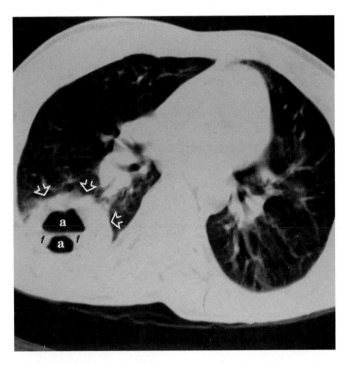

Figure 3–30 Lung abscess. A PA chest radiograph shows an irregularly thick-walled cavitary mass lesion in the right lower lobe (arrows).

Figure 3–31 Lung abscess. A CT scan of the same patient as in Figure 3–30 shows lobulated abscess margins (open arrows) and air-fluid levels within the abscess cavity (**a** represents air; **f**, fluid).

3.14 LUNG NODULES

3.14.1 Solitary Pulmonary Nodules

A common occurrence in a busy emergency room is the finding of a solitary pulmonary nodule on a chest radiograph. Many of these nodules turn out to be artifacts created by superimposed structures. The differential diagnosis of a solitary pulmonary nodule includes both primary and metastatic malignancies, granulomas (tuberculosis, histoplasmosis), benign neoplasms (adenomas, hamartomas), infections, pulmonary arteriovenous malformations, and pulmonary infarcts. Chest radiography and CT are the two modalities used for evaluating solitary nodules.

Chest radiography is a useful but insensitive screening modality for pulmonary nodules. Nodules smaller than 1 cm are usually not detected with plain film radiography. Furthermore, the error rate for the detection of early lung cancer has been reported to be as high as 50%. Once a nodule has been found and confirmed with oblique radiographs, a CT scan of the chest should be performed.

Chest CT is the most sensitive imaging modality for evaluating lung nodules, and allows identification of characteristics (ie, benign-appearing central calcifications, smooth versus spiculated margins) that help in narrowing the differential diagnosis. Furthermore, other nodules not seen on chest radiographs may become more apparent. Simultaneous evaluation for mediastinal adenopathy and tumor staging can also be performed. CT-guided biopsies of solitary nodules may avoid the need for an open lung biopsy and thoracotomy.

3.14.2 Multiple Pulmonary Nodules

Metastatic disease is the most common cause of multiple pulmonary nodules. The most common primary tumors resulting in lung metastases are breast, thyroid, gastrointestinal tract, and testicular malignancies in adults, and Wilms' tumor, Ewing's sarcoma, neuroblastoma and osteosarcoma in children. These nodules are usually found in the lower lobes, and occur more commonly in the lung periphery. Other causes of multiple pulmonary nodules include infections, septic emboli, Wegener's granulomatosis, rheumatoid arthritis, and arteriovenous malformations (hereditary hemorrhagic telangiectasia syndrome).

As with solitary pulmonary nodules, chest radiography and CT are the two best imaging modalities; however, chest CT has superior sensitivity. Nodules appear as multiple round densities of varying sizes. Mediastinal involvement can be evaluated and the differential diagnosis narrowed by specific characteristics of the lesions. Very large round lesions, referred to as "cannon ball" lesions, are classically seen with colonic metastasis. Thyroid metastases usually present as multiple small lesions.

SELECTED REFERENCES

Caskey CI, Templeton PA, Zerhouni EA. Current evaluation of the solitary pulmonary nodule. Radiol Clin North Am. 1990; 28: 511–520.

Midthun DE, Swensen SJ, Jett JR. Clinical strategies for solitary pulmonary nodule. Annu Rev Med. 1992; 43: 195–208.

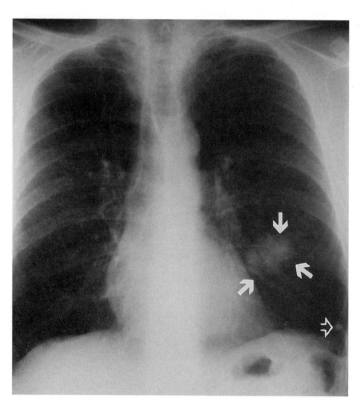

Figure 3–32 Pulmonary nodule. Radiograph of the chest reveals a well-circumscribed mass in the left lung base (arrows). A small peripheral granuloma is also noted (open arrow).

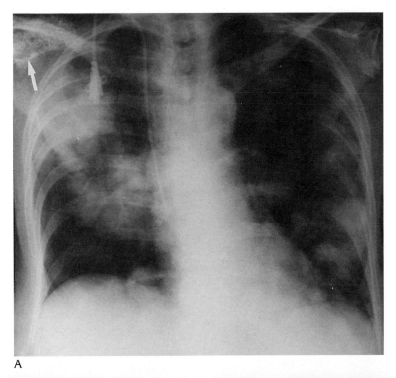

A

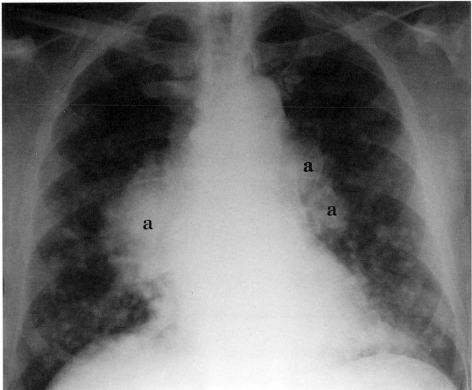

B

Figure 3–33A, B Multiple pulmonary nodules.   Radiographs of two patients with multiple pulmonary nodules due to metastatic renal cell carcinoma (**A**) and metastatic thyroid carcinoma (**B**). Note the osteolytic lesion of the right scapula in **A** (arrow) and extensive mediastinal adenopathy (**a**) in **B**.

3.15 PNEUMOTHORAX

A pneumothorax represents a collection of air between the visceral and parietal pleura, resulting in passive atelectasis of the adjacent lung. Pneumothoraces most commonly result from penetrating trauma or blunt trauma with pleural damage caused by an associated rib fracture. Spontaneous pneumothorax is a rare entity seen in young thin males, usually owing to rupture of congenital subpleural bullae. Other less common causes include asthma, chronic obstructive lung disease, interstitial lung diseases (eg, lymphangioleiomyomatosis, cystic fibrosis, histiocytosis X), catamenial pneumothorax (pleural endometriosis), necrotizing pneumonia with bronchopleural fistula formation, after lung biopsy or thoracentesis, positive pressure mechanical ventilation, esophageal perforation, and malignancy (eg, metastatic osteosarcoma). Patients complain of a stabbing pleuritic type chest pain on the affected side and dyspnea as a consequence of splinting and atelectasis. The diagnosis is usually made by a chest radiograph that shows a collection of air in the pleural space. Since this air is fixed in volume relative to the lung, the pneumothorax appears larger on films obtained in expiration. When air in the pleural space accumulates under pressure, a tension pneumothorax occurs, with the potential for respiratory and circulatory compromise because of compression of the lung, inversion of the diaphragm, mediastinal shift, and restriction of venous return to the right atrium. Treatment is decompression of the pneumothorax by insertion of one or multiple chest tubes. For small or iatrogenically induced pneumothoraces, the fluoroscopic insertion of small-bore tubes is generally sufficient for complete expansion of the affected lung. The chest tubes can be removed when the pneumothorax and any associated air leak are resolved. Pleurodesis using the intrapleural administration of bleomycin or talc may prevent recurrences.

SELECTED REFERENCES

Sassoon CS. The etiology and treatment of spontaneous pneumothorax. Curr Opin Pulm Med. 1995; 1: 331–338.

Spillane RM, Shepard JO, Deluca SA. Radiographic aspects of pneumothorax. Am Fam Physician. 1995; 51: 459–464.

Light RW, Vargas FS. Pleural sclerosis for the treatment of pneumothorax and pleural effusion. Lung. 1997; 175: 213–223.

Walker-Renard PB, Vaughan LM, Sahn SA. Chemical pleurodesis for malignant pleural effusions. Ann Intern Med. 1994; 120: 56–64.

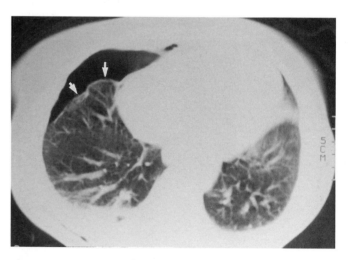

Figure 3–35 Pneumothorax. CT scan showing the pleural margin (arrows) and collection of air within the pleural space. CT is highly sensitive for the detection of small pneumothoraces.

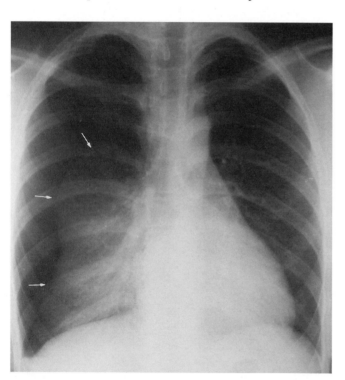

Figure 3–34 Pneumothorax. Chest radiograph reveals no vessels extending beyond the edge of the visualized visceral pleural reflection (arrows). Mild, passive atelectasis of the remaining air-filled lung is seen.

3.16 RIB FRACTURES AND LUNG CONTUSION

Rib fractures are commonly seen in the emergency room setting. They can be well assessed using a "rib series" consisting of multiple oblique radiographs of the rib cage. In the trauma setting, rib fractures have almost no clinical significance and do not alter the patient's management, although an associated pneumothorax or lung contusion should be evaluated for with a chest radiograph. Primary bone tumors, metastatic tumors to the bone, and benign bone lesions may result in the development of "pathologic" rib fractures despite only minimal trauma. In such cases, radionuclide bone scans or CT with bone windows are much more sensitive than radiographs for the detection of underlying abnormalities of the rib. Common primary neoplasms that metastasize to bone and subsequently result in pathologic fractures include lung cancer, breast cancer, prostate cancer, and renal cancer.

A displaced fracture is easily seen on chest radiography as an abrupt interruption in the rib contour. A nondisplaced fracture is more difficult to recognize, although a surrounding hematoma represented by a plueral opacity with obtuse margins may be seen adjacent to the involved rib. Occasionally, fractures may not be evident until delayed radiographs (10 days to 2 weeks) reveal callous formation. In contrast, both displaced and nondisplaced rib fractures are easily identified by CT and appear as linear defects through the cortex of the bone with an associated hematoma.

The most common pulmonary complication of blunt chest trauma is the development of intraparenchymal hemorrhage referred to as a lung contusion. On a chest radiograph, this can appear as a focal opacity in the lung or may assume an "alveolar edema pattern." This latter pattern refers to the appearance of multifocal ill-defined densities within the lung parenchyma. Associated rib fractures overlying the contusion are common. The opacification is seldom symmetric with greater involvement on the side of maximum impact. These radiographic changes are seen soon after trauma and resolve rapidly over the course of the next 1 to 7 days.

On CT, pulmonary contusions appear as focal infiltrates. Rib fractures and pleural effusions are also commonly seen. The contusion begins to clear very rapidly within the first 24 to 48 hours.

SELECTED REFERENCES

Wagner RB, Slivko B, Jamieson PM. Effect of lung contusion on pulmonary hemodynamics. Ann Thorac Surg. 1991; 52: 5–57.

Cohn SM. Pulmonary contusion: review of the clinical entity. J Trauma. 1997; 42: 973–979.

Allen GS, Coates NE. Pulmonary contusion: a collective review. Am Surg. 1996; 62: 895–900.

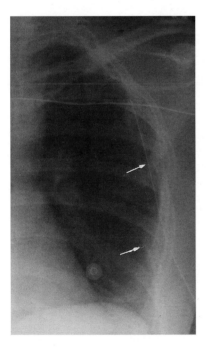

Figure 3–36 Rib fractures. Chest film of a patient who sustained blunt trauma to the left side of the chest during a motor vehicle accident. Multiple fractures of the posterior and lateral ribs on the left side are evident by disruption in the normal bony cortex (arrows). A chest tube has been inserted to treat an associated pneumothorax.

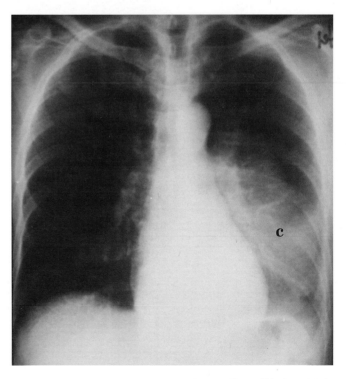

Figure 3–37 Pulmonary contusion. Consolidation (c) is noted in the left lower lobe following a motor vehicle accident. This was noted to clear quickly on subsequent radiographs.

3.17 PLEURAL EFFUSION AND HEMOTHORAX

Fluid collections within the pleural space are either transudates (caused by altered hydrostatic pressures) or exudates (resulting from increased permeability or trauma). Transudative effusions occur secondary to congestive heart failure, hypoalbuminemia, volume overload, or extension of abdominal fluid collections. Causes of exudative effusions include pulmonary infections, malignancy, pulmonary embolism, collagen-vascular disease, trauma, and inflammatory conditions (eg, Dressler's syndrome). An effusion is considered a hemothorax when the hematocrit of the pleural fluid is >20%. Malignancy is suspected when a sanguinous effusion is present in the absence of trauma, and cytologic examinations are positive in approximately 60% (after examination of a single thoracentesis specimen) to 80% (with evaluation of several specimens). Radiographs of the chest will show blunting of the lateral or posterior costophrenic sulci and increased opacity representing the effusion. Decubitus films are useful for identifying smaller effusions and show whether the fluid is freely mobile within the pleural space. Careful examination should be performed to evaluate for cardiomegaly, lymphadenopathy, pleural or parenchymal masses, infiltrates, rib lesions, abdominal disease, or other underlying causes of the effusion. Ultrasonography or CT may allow recognition of the pleural fluid and guide percutaneous drainage of loculated collections and hemothoraces. Chemical pleurodesis using the intrapleural administration of bleomycin or talc is effective in reducing or eliminating the recurrent accumulation of malignant effusions in approximately 85% of cases.

SELECTED REFERENCES

Yeam I, Sassoon C. Hemothorax and chylothorax. Curr Opin Pulm Med. 1997; 3: 310–314.

Martinez FJ, Villanueva AG, Pickering R, et al. Spontaneous hemothorax. Report of 6 cases and review of the literature. Medicine (Baltimore). 1992; 71: 354–368.

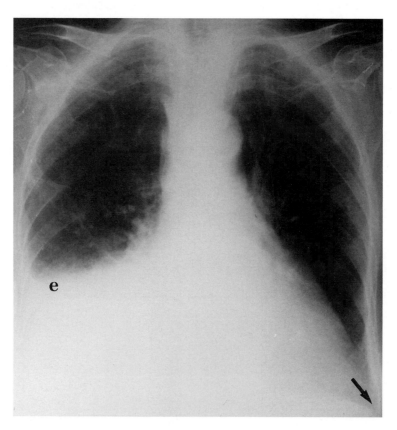

Figure 3–38 Pleural effusion. Chest radiograph shows blunting of the right costophrenic angle and increased density at the right lung base resulting from layering of a pleural effusion (**e**). The left costophrenic sulcus is sharply delineated (arrow).

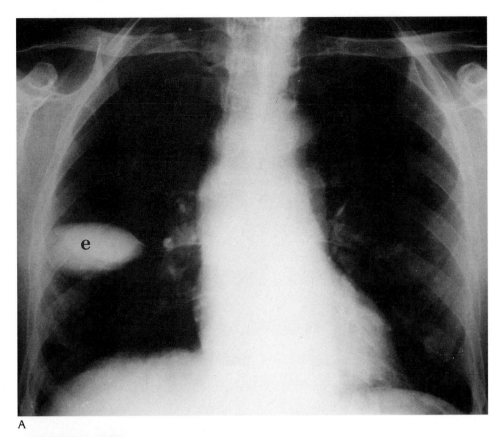

A

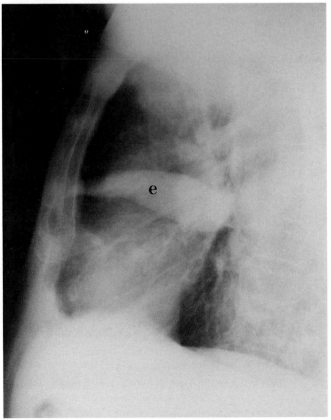

B

Figure 3–39A, B Loculated pleural effusion. Posteroanterior (**A**) and lateral (**B**) chest radiographs reveal a lenticular density in the mid chest on the right side. The lateral film confirms this to be a pseudotumor caused by accumulation of pleural fluid (**e**) within the minor fissure on the right side.

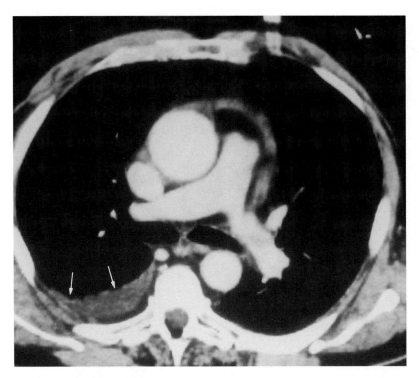

Figure 3–40 Pleural effusion. CT scan showing small freely layering pleural effusion (arrows) on the right side. CT is the most sensitive examination for detecting pleural fluid collections.

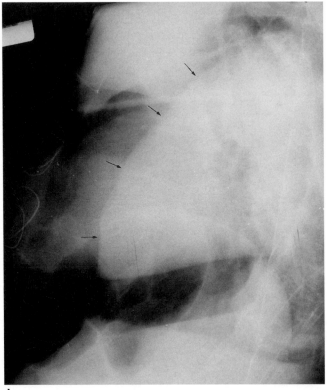

A

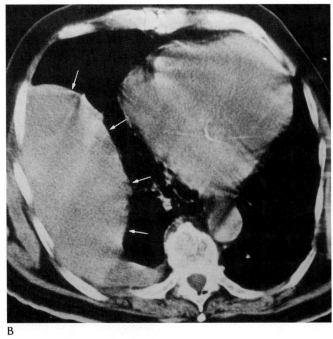

B

Figure 3–41A, B Hemothorax. Lateral chest film (**A**) and CT scan (**B**) showing a loculated high-density pleural fluid collection (arrows) in a patient receiving coumadin anticoagulation for a prosthetic heart valve. Percutaneous drainage proved the collection to be a hemothorax.

3.18 DIAPHRAGMATIC RUPTURE

Traumatic rupture of the diaphragm usually results from blunt or penetrating trauma to the abdomen but can also occur with trauma to the thorax. The left hemidiaphragm is involved in more than 90% of the cases, and ruptures of the central or posterior diaphragm are the most frequent. As a result, intra-abdominal viscera may herniate into the chest cavity. The stomach is the organ most frequently herniated, but omentum, spleen, small or large intestine, liver, and kidney may all herniate into the chest. Occasionally, delayed herniation may occur days to weeks after the diaphragmatic rupture.

The radiographic signs vary with the extent of the rupture, depending upon which organs herniated through the injured diaphragm, and whether the herniated organs contain air or are fluid filled. There may be apparent elevation of the hemidiaphragm if fluid filled or solid organ herniation is present. A change in shape and position of the apparent dome of the diaphragm is strongly suggestive of traumatic herniation. Absence of the normal gastric air bubble and discernible bowel shadows in the thorax may make the diagnosis obvious. The administration of barium by mouth and by rectum helps identify the relationship of the bowel to the diaphragm.

CT can be helpful in diagnosing traumatic diaphragmatic ruptures. Bowel or viscera or both are seen in the thorax due to the disrupted diaphragm. Coronal reconstructions facilitate recognition of any herniated abdomen organs. Since MRI scans may be obtained in the coronal plane, it is an ideal modality for studying diaphragmatic ruptures. Ultrasound has limited utility but may detect large defects in the diaphragm.

SELECTED REFERENCES

Shackleton KL, Stewart ET, Taylor AJ. Traumatic diaphragmatic injuries: spectrum of radiographic findings. Radiographics. 1998; 18: 49–59.

Shah R, Sabanathan S, Mearns AJ, Choudhury AK. Traumatic rupture of the diaphragm. Ann Thorac Surg. 1995; 60: 1444–1449.

Murray JG, Caoili E, Gruden JF, et al. Acute rupture of the diaphragm due to blunt trauma: diagnostic sensitivity and specificity of CT. AJR. 1996; 166: 1035–1039.

Kim HH, Shin YR, Kim KJ, et al. Blunt traumatic rupture of the diaphragm: sonographic diagnosis. J Ultrasound Med. 1997; 16: 593–598.

Gelman R, Virvis SE, Gens D. Diaphragmatic rupture due to blunt trauma: sensitivity of plain chest radiographs. AJR. 1991; 156: 51–57.

Shapiro MJ, Heiberg E, Durham RM, et al. The unreliability of CT scans and initial chest radiographs in evaluating blunt trauma induced diaphragmatic rupture. Clin Radiol. 1996; 51: 27–30.

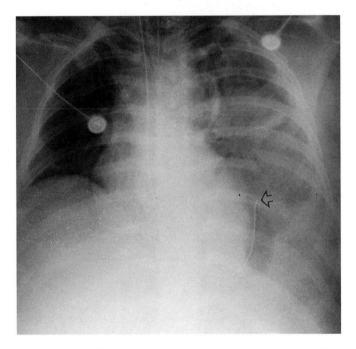

Figure 3–42 Diaphragmatic rupture. Radiograph of the chest shows increased opacity at the left lung base and loss of the normal diaphragmatic shadow. The tip of the nasogastric tube (open arrow) points upward toward the body of the stomach, which is within the left side of the chest.

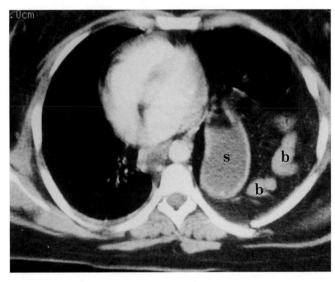

Figure 3–43 Diaphragmatic rupture. CT scan at the lung bases in the same patient as in Figure 3–42 shows the stomach (**s**) and several small bowel loops (**b**) in the left hemithorax.

3.19 PERICARDIAL EFFUSION

Pericardial effusions may be idiopathic or may occur in association with fluid overload, hypoalbuminemia, trauma, aortic dissection, neoplasms, and many other conditions causing pericarditis. Sudden accumulations of fluid or blood in the pericardial space may result in hemodynamic instability (pericardial tamponade), whereas collections accumulating slowly may be tolerated with minimal signs and symptoms. Although echocardiography is the definitive diagnostic examination, a chest film may show enlargement of the cardiac silhouette with a "water-bottle" configuration. Therapy for acute tamponade is fluid resuscitation, inotropic support, and prompt pericardio-centesis. More chronic effusions are managed by treatment of the underlying cause of pericarditis.

SELECTED REFERENCES

Vaitkus PT, Herrmann HC, LeWinter MM. Treatment of malignant pericardial effusion. JAMA. 1994; 272: 59–64.

Chong HH, Plotnick GD. Pericardial effusion and tamponade: evaluation, imaging modalities, and management. Compr Ther. 1995; 21: 378–385.

Fowler NO. Cardiac tamponade. A clinical or an echocardiographic diagnosis? Circulation. 1993; 87: 1738–1741.

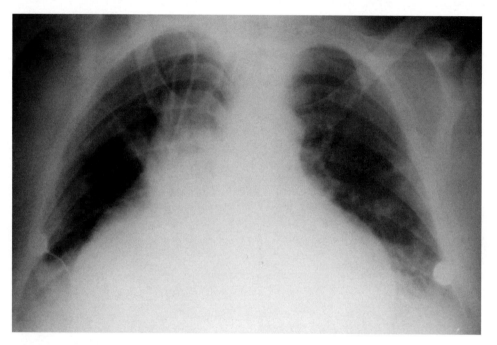

Figure 3–44 Pericardial effusion. Chest film showing the characteristic "water-bottle" configuration of the cardiac silhouette.

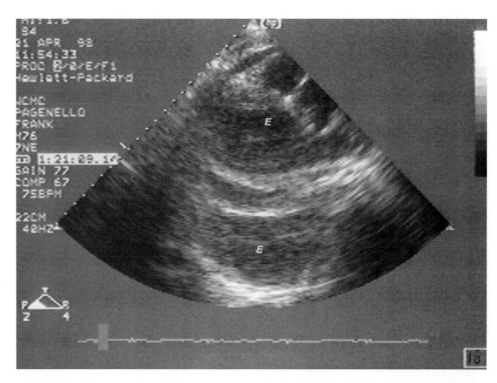

Figure 3–45 Pericardial effusion.   Long axis parasternal view revealing anterior and posterior echo-free spaces consistent with a circumferential pericardial effusion (**E**).

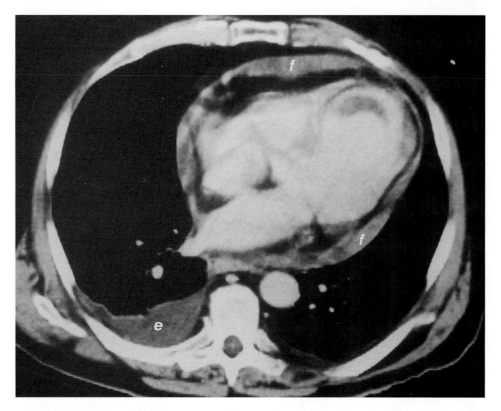

Figure 3–46 Pericardial effusion.   CT scan of a patient with pericarditis. Fluid within the pericardial sac is seen (**f**) as well as a small pleural effusion on the right side (**e**).

3.20 PNEUMOMEDIASTINUM

A pneumomediastinum is the collection of air within the mediastinal space. Although this air collection is itself benign, the presence of a pneumomediastinum may be the harbinger of serious underlying disease. Causes of pneumomediastinum include closed chest trauma, rupture of the esophagus, bronchial or tracheal tears, parenchymal injury to the lung, asthma, and extension of gas from below the diaphragm or from the cervical region.

On chest radiographs, the heart shadow normally silhouettes and obscures the medial aspect of the diaphragm. A pneumomediastinum causes a characteristic interposition of gas between the heart and the diaphragm that permits visualization of the medial aspect of the diaphragm. This has been termed the "continuous diaphragm" sign. Elevation of the mediastinal pleura along the left side of the heart border is another radiographic finding of a pneumomediastinum. In newborns and young children, the mediastinal air surrounds and lifts the relatively large thymus, producing the "angel's wings" sign. CT will identify a pneumomediastinum not seen on chest radiographs as black areas within the mediastinum.

SELECTED REFERENCES

Smith BA, Fergusion DB. Disposition of spontaneous pneumomediastinum. Am J Emerg Med. 1991; 9: 256–259.

Bejvan SM, Godwin JD. Pneumomediastinum: old signs and new signs. AJR. 1996; 166: 1041–1048.

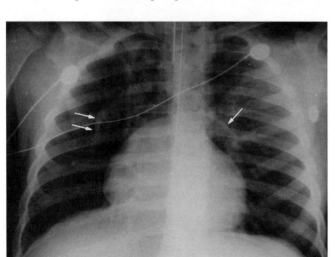

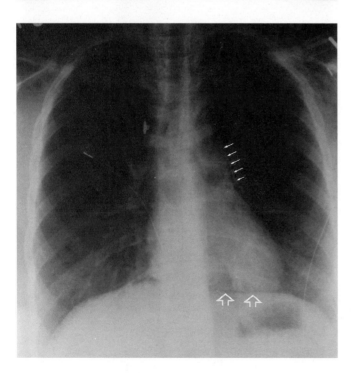

Figure 3–47 Pneumomediastinum in a young child. An "angel wings" sign is seen as a result of elevation of the thymus (arrows) by air in the mediastinal space.

Figure 3–48 Pneumomediastinum in an adult. A thin lucent stripe (small arrows) is seen adjacent to the heart border on the left side as a result of mediastinal air. Air outlining the medial aspect of the left hemidiaphragm (open arrows) produces the "continuous diaphragm" sign.

3.21 FOREIGN BODY ASPIRATION

Obstruction of a major airway by a foreign body occurs more commonly in children. The resulting ball-valve type of obstruction as well as collateral air drift causes air-trapping in the affected lung that appears on radiographs as hyperinflation, hyperlucency, and mediastinal shift. Owing to the relatively fixed volume of the affected side relative to the contralateral lung, these x-ray findings are more pronounced in films obtained during expiration. In adults, collateral air drift is less prevalent, and occlusion of a major airway is more likely to result in a pattern of postobstructive atelectasis and volume loss. Occasionally, acute airway obstruction may cause noncardiogenic pulmonary edema with roentgenographic evidence of pulmonary venous hypertension and diffuse alveolar infiltration. Bronchoscopy is both diagnostic and frequently therapeutic, and surgery is rarely necessary to remove the aspirated foreign body.

SELECTED REFERENCES

Losek JD. Diagnostic difficulties of foreign body aspiration in children. Am J Emerg Med. 1990; 8: 348–350.

Aboussouan LS, Stoller JK. Diagnosis and management of upper airway obstruction. Clin Chest Med. 1994; 15: 35–53.

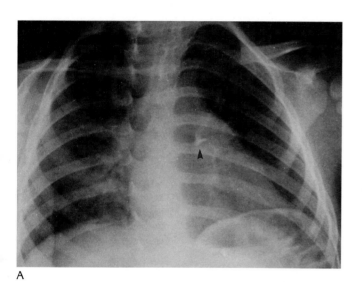

A

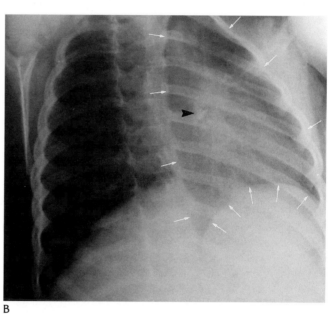

B

Figure 3–49A, B Foreign body aspiration.   Radiographs of the chest obtained in AP (**A**) and left lateral decubitus (**B**) positions reveals air-trapping and hyperlucency of the dependent left lung (outlined in arrows). Normally, the dependent lung on a decubitus film appears compressed. An aspirated radiopaque foreign body (**A, B**) is seen (arrowhead).

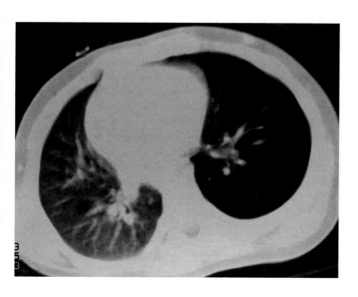

Figure 3–50 Foreign body aspiration.   CT scan of the same patient as in Figure 3-49. Air-trapping and increased lucency of the left hemithorax is readily apparent. Note the compensatory redistribution of pulmonary circulation to the right side.

CHAPTER 4

ABDOMEN AND PELVIS IMAGING

John H. Rundback, MD

Maurice R. Poplausky, MD

Bok Y. Lee, MD, FACS

4.1 NORMALS

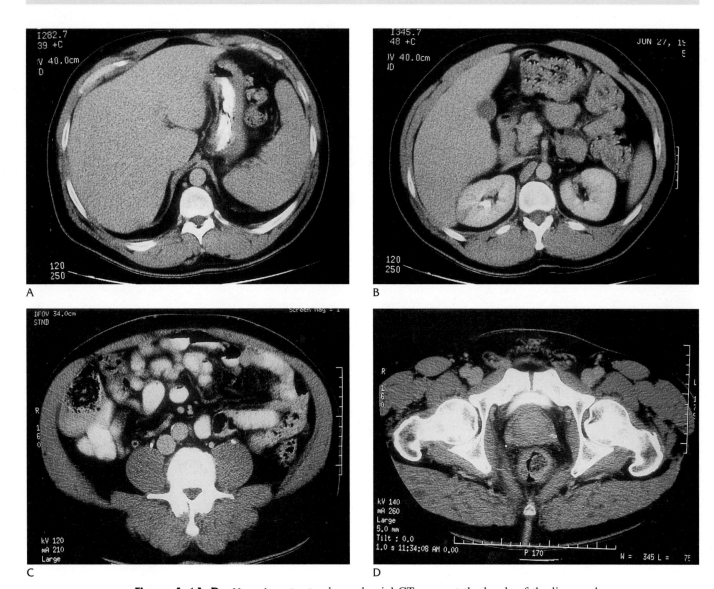

Figure 4–1A–D Normal contrast-enhanced axial CT scans at the levels of the liver and spleen (**A**), see opposite page; kidneys (**B**), see page 84; lower abdomen (**C**), see page 85; and pelvis (**D**), see page 86.

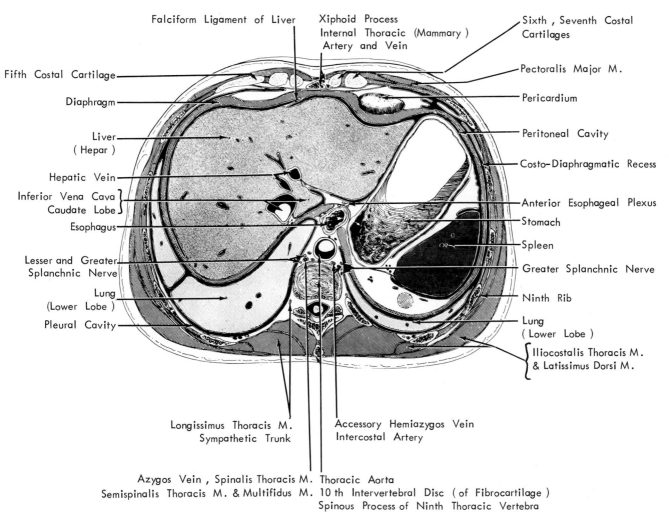

Falciform Ligament of Liver

Xiphoid Process
Internal Thoracic (Mammary)
Artery and Vein

Sixth, Seventh Costal
Cartilages

Fifth Costal Cartilage

Diaphragm

Liver
(Hepar)

Hepatic Vein
Inferior Vena Cava
Caudate Lobe
Esophagus

Lesser and Greater
Splanchnic Nerve

Lung
(Lower Lobe)
Pleural Cavity

Pectoralis Major M.

Pericardium

Peritoneal Cavity

Costo-Diaphragmatic Recess

Anterior Esophageal Plexus
Stomach
Spleen

Greater Splanchnic Nerve

Ninth Rib

Lung
(Lower Lobe)

Iliocostalis Thoracis M.
& Latissimus Dorsi M.

Longissimus Thoracis M.
Sympathetic Trunk

Accessory Hemiazygos Vein
Intercostal Artery

Azygos Vein, Spinalis Thoracis M.
Semispinalis Thoracis M. & Multifidus M.

Thoracic Aorta
10 th Intervertebral Disc (of Fibrocartilage)
Spinous Process of Ninth Thoracic Vertebra

E

Figure 4–1E–H Sectional drawings, corresponding to Figures 4–1A–D, show normal anatomic structures.

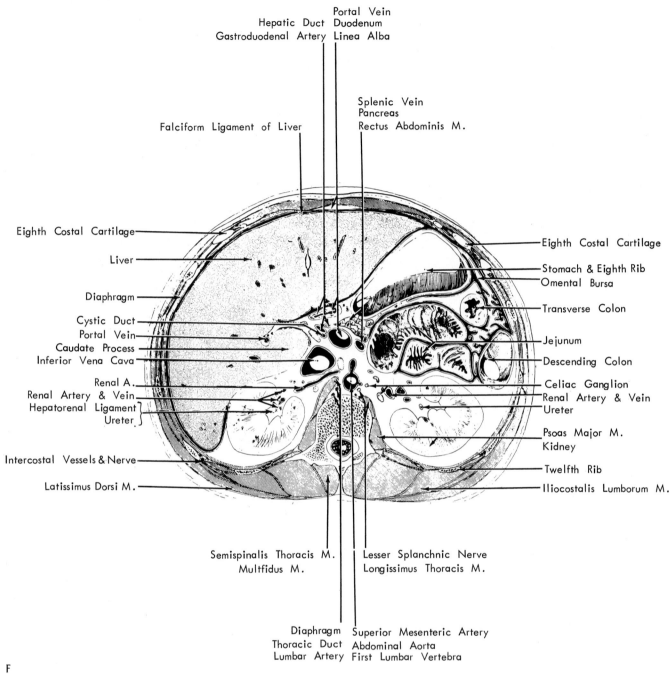

Portal Vein
Hepatic Duct Duodenum
Gastroduodenal Artery Linea Alba

Splenic Vein
Pancreas
Rectus Abdominis M.

Falciform Ligament of Liver

Eighth Costal Cartilage

Liver

Diaphragm

Cystic Duct
Portal Vein
Caudate Process
Inferior Vena Cava

Renal A.
Renal Artery & Vein
Hepatorenal Ligament
Ureter

Intercostal Vessels & Nerve

Latissimus Dorsi M.

Eighth Costal Cartilage

Stomach & Eighth Rib
Omental Bursa

Transverse Colon

Jejunum

Descending Colon

Celiac Ganglion
Renal Artery & Vein
Ureter

Psoas Major M.
Kidney

Twelfth Rib

Iliocostalis Lumborum M.

Semispinalis Thoracis M.
Multfidus M.

Lesser Splanchnic Nerve
Longissimus Thoracis M.

Diaphragm
Thoracic Duct
Lumbar Artery

Superior Mesenteric Artery
Abdominal Aorta
First Lumbar Vertebra

F

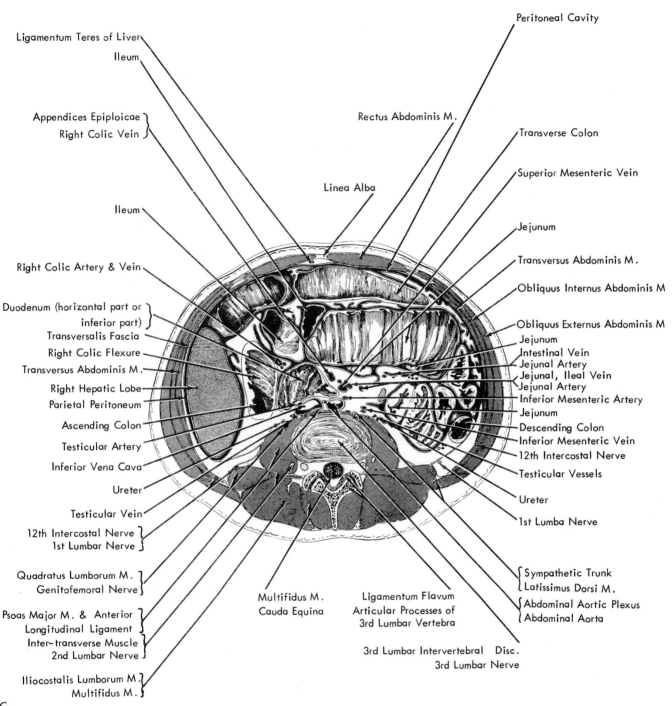

Ligamentum Teres of Liver
Ileum

Appendices Epiploicae
Right Colic Vein

Ileum

Right Colic Artery & Vein

Duodenum (horizontal part or
inferior part)
Transversalis Fascia
Right Colic Flexure
Transversus Abdominis M.
Right Hepatic Lobe
Parietal Peritoneum
Ascending Colon
Testicular Artery
Inferior Vena Cava
Ureter
Testicular Vein
12th Intercostal Nerve
1st Lumbar Nerve

Quadratus Lumborum M.
Genitofemoral Nerve

Psoas Major M. & Anterior
Longitudinal Ligament
Inter-transverse Muscle
2nd Lumbar Nerve

Iliocostalis Lumborum M.
Multifidus M.

Peritoneal Cavity

Rectus Abdominis M.

Linea Alba

Transverse Colon

Superior Mesenteric Vein

Jejunum

Transversus Abdominis M.

Obliquus Internus Abdominis M

Obliquus Externus Abdominis M
Jejunum
Intestinal Vein
Jejunal Artery
Jejunal, Ileal Vein
Jejunal Artery
Inferior Mesenteric Artery
Jejunum
Descending Colon
Inferior Mesenteric Vein
12th Intercostal Nerve
Testicular Vessels
Ureter
1st Lumba Nerve

Sympathetic Trunk
Latissimus Dorsi M.
Abdominal Aortic Plexus
Abdominal Aorta

Multifidus M.
Cauda Equina

Ligamentum Flavum
Articular Processes of
3rd Lumbar Vertebra

3rd Lumbar Intervertebral Disc.
3rd Lumbar Nerve

G

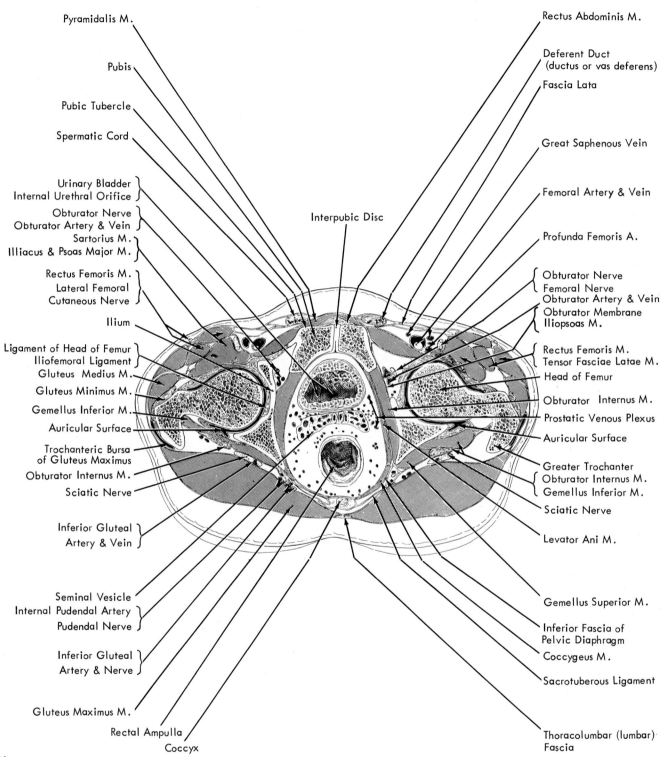

Pyramidalis M.

Pubis

Pubic Tubercle

Spermatic Cord

Urinary Bladder
Internal Urethral Orifice
Obturator Nerve
Obturator Artery & Vein
Sartorius M.
Illiacus & Psoas Major M.

Rectus Femoris M.
Lateral Femoral
Cutaneous Nerve

Ilium

Ligament of Head of Femur
Iliofemoral Ligament
Gluteus Medius M.

Gluteus Minimus M.

Gemellus Inferior M.

Auricular Surface

Trochanteric Bursa
of Gluteus Maximus

Obturator Internus M.

Sciatic Nerve

Inferior Gluteal
Artery & Vein

Seminal Vesicle
Internal Pudendal Artery
Pudendal Nerve

Inferior Gluteal
Artery & Nerve

Gluteus Maximus M.

Rectal Ampulla

Coccyx

Interpubic Disc

Rectus Abdominis M.

Deferent Duct
(ductus or vas deferens)

Fascia Lata

Great Saphenous Vein

Femoral Artery & Vein

Profunda Femoris A.

Obturator Nerve
Femoral Nerve
Obturator Artery & Vein
Obturator Membrane
Iliopsoas M.

Rectus Femoris M.
Tensor Fasciae Latae M.

Head of Femur

Obturator Internus M.

Prostatic Venous Plexus

Auricular Surface

Greater Trochanter
Obturator Internus M.
Gemellus Inferior M.

Sciatic Nerve

Levator Ani M.

Gemellus Superior M.

Inferior Fascia of
Pelvic Diaphragm

Coccygeus M.

Sacrotuberous Ligament

Thoracolumbar (lumbar)
Fascia

H

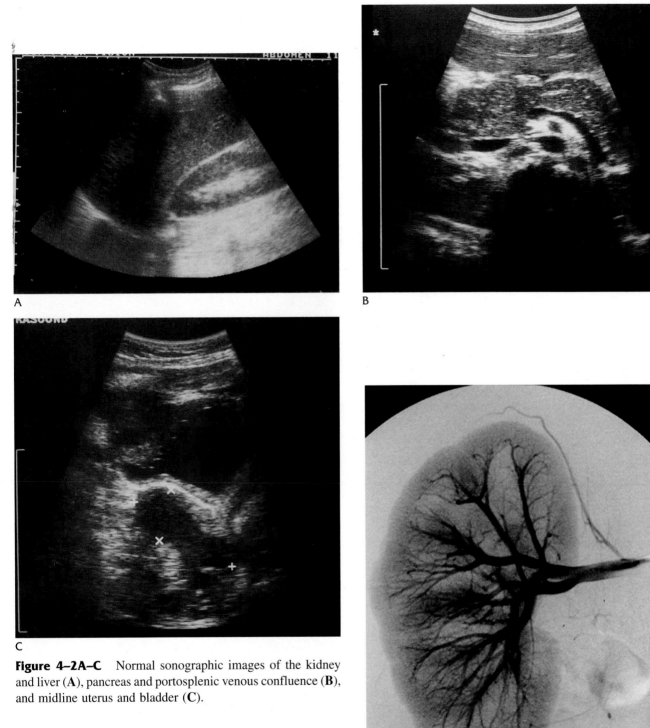

Figure 4–2A–C Normal sonographic images of the kidney and liver (**A**), pancreas and portosplenic venous confluence (**B**), and midline uterus and bladder (**C**).

Figure 4–3 Normal selective right renal arteriogram, late arterial phase.

4.2 ABDOMINAL AORTIC ANEURYSM

The normal abdominal aorta measures up to 3 cm in diameter and progressively tapers as it proceeds distally. If the abdominal aorta measures more than 3 cm or fails to taper, an aneurysm is present. Atherosclerosis is responsible for >90% of abdominal aortic aneurysms (AAAs), although an abnormality in connective tissue metabolism has been implicated in their etiology. Atherosclerotic aneurysms most commonly arise below the renal artery origins, and mural calcification outlining the aneurysm sac is detectable on plain radiographs in most cases. Seventy percent of patients with AAAs are symptomatic; the most common symptom is abdominal pain (37%) or a pulsatile mass (26%). The major risk of untreated AAAs is aneurysm rupture, which is directly proportional to aneurysm size. For aneurysms measuring 4 cm in diameter, the lifetime risk of rupture is 7%; for aneurysms >5 cm in diameter, this lifetime risk increases to almost 25%. Indications for surgical repair include a diameter >5 cm, an increase in diameter of >0.5 cm over a 6-month period, an overall increase in diameter of 1.0 cm during any period of observation, or symptoms related to the aneurysm.

Other complications of AAAs include spontaneous dissection, branch vessel occlusion with resultant renal or mesenteric ischemia, pain from local mass effect, peripheral embolization, secondary infection, and acute aortic occlusion.

Since mural thrombus may lead to an underestimation of aneurysm diameter by angiography, aneurysm size is best measured using abdominal sonography or computed tomography. CT angiography with 3-D reconstruction is an excellent way to view an abdominal aortic aneurysm because the relationship of the aneurysm to branch vessels can be well seen. Angiography is no longer used to diagnose AAA. It is, however, an essential part of the preoperative evaluation and is used to evaluate the relationship of the aneurysm to the renal arteries, to determine the patency of the visceral and iliac vessels, and to detect aberrant vessels.

Percutaneously introduced stent grafts have recently been approved for the treatment of AAAs and are an alternative to open surgery in selected cases.

SELECTED REFERENCES

Pleumeekers HJCM, Hoes AW, van der Does E, et al. Epidemiology of abdominal aortic aneurysms. Eur J Vasc Surg. 1994; 8: 119–128.

Errington ML, Ferguson JM, Gillespie IN, et al. Complete pre-operative imaging assessment of abdominal aortic aneurysm with spiral CT angiography. Clin Radiol. 1997; 52: 369–377.

Sardelic F, Fletcher JP, Ho D, Simmons K. Assessment of abdominal aortic aneurysm with magnetic resonance imaging. Australas Radiol. 1995; 39: 107–111.

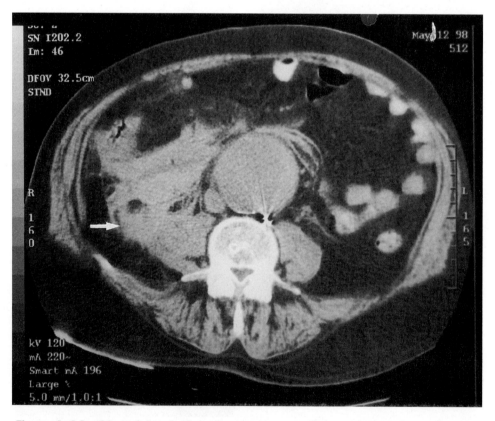

Figure 4–4 Leaking abdominal aortic aneurysm. CT scan shows a 7-cm infrarenal abdominal aortic aneurysm. There is extensive infiltration of the retroperitoneal fat by hemorrhage (arrow).

4.3 INFLAMMATORY ANEURYSM

Inflammatory aneurysms of the abdominal aorta account for approximately 3–5% of all abdominal aneurysms, and are characterized by thickening of the aortic wall and a perianeurysmal inflammatory reaction consisting of an extensive mononuclear lymphocytic infiltration. Their origin is uncertain. A characteristic triad of abdominal or back pain, elevation of the erythrocyte sedimentation rate, and weight loss are present in only 22% of cases. Obstruction of the ureters and involvement of the duodenum may also occur. On CT and MRI, a thick mantle of soft tissue involving the anterior and lateral aorta with sparing of the posterior aspect of the aorta is noted; ureteral obstruction with hydronephrosis may also be identified. Angiography shows the size and extent of the aneurysm, and multiple aneurysms may occasionally be seen. Immunosuppressive therapy should be used with caution because it may increase the risk of aortic rupture. Aneurysm resection is associated with regression of the inflammatory process in two thirds of cases.

SELECTED REFERENCES

Rasmussen TE, Hallett JW. Inflammatory aortic aneurysms: a clinical review with new perspectives in pathogenesis. Ann Surg. 1997; 225: 155–164.

Mauro MA. Inflammatory abdominal aortic aneurysm. Abdom Imaging. 1997; 22: 357–358.

Hayashi H, Kumazaki T. Case report: inflammatory abdominal aortic aneurysm—dynamic GD-DTPA enhanced magnetic resonance imaging features. Br J Radiol. 1995; 68: 321–323.

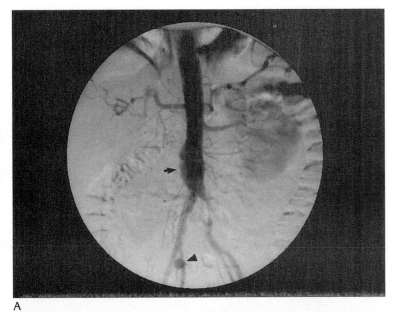

A

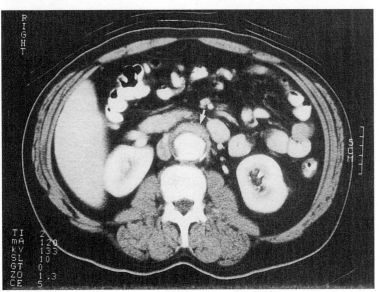

B

Figure 4–5A, B Inflammatory aneurysm. An abdominal aortogram (**A**) shows an irregular, lobulated aneurysm above the aortic bifurcation (arrow). There is a second small aneurysm of the right hypogastric artery (arrowhead). A CT image (**B**) of the same patient reveals a thick mantle of inflammatory tissue anterior and lateral to the aorta (arrow).

4.4 ABDOMINAL AORTIC DISSECTION

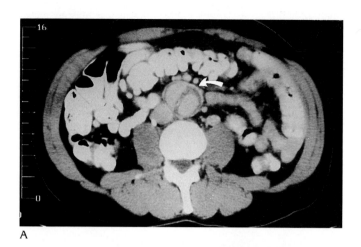

A

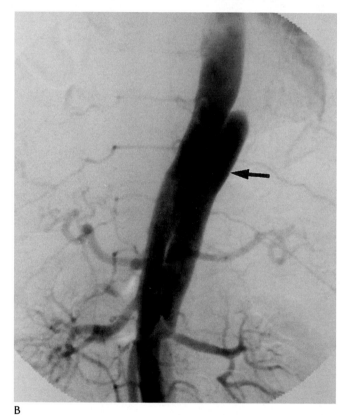

B

Figure 4–6A, B Abdominal aortic dissection. A contrast-enhanced CT scan (**A**) reveals a dilated mid-abdominal aorta. Note the separation of the true and false lumina by a thick nonenhancing intimal flap (curved arrow). An abdominal aortogram (**B**) in the same patient clearly displays contrast within both lumens. The false lumen is on the patient's left side (arrow).

Dissection of the abdominal aorta most commonly occurs as an extension of a type 2 or type 3 thoracic aortic dissection. However, isolated spontaneous involvement of the abdominal aorta from undermining and dehiscence of an ulcerated atheromatous plaque has been described. Dissection may also be trau-

matic or iatrogenic, occurring after attempted catheterization, thrombectomy, or endarterectomy. Regardless of the cause, potential complications include: (1) visceral or lumbar branch vessel occlusion (with resulting renal or mesenteric ischemia), (2) aortoiliac thrombosis, (3) acute lower limb ischemia, (4) aortic rupture, and (5) delayed aneurysmal dilatation. Cross-sectional imaging including computed tomography (CT), CT angiography (CTA) with 3-D reconstruction, and MRI characteristically reveal an intimal flap separating the true and false lumina. Periaortic hematoma is indicative of acute aortic leakage and mandates urgent surgical intervention. Angiography is critical in operative cases for showing the extent of the aortic dissection and involvement of the visceral or iliac arteries. Percutaneous treatments, including septal fenestration of the dissection flap and endovascular stenting of the aortic lumen or compromised branch vessels, may allow definitive management in selected patients.

SELECTED REFERENCES

Williams DM, Lee DY, Hamilton BH, et al. The dissected aorta: percutaneous treatment of ischemic complications—principles and results. J Vasc Interv Radiol. 1997; 8: 605–625.

Becquemin JP, Deleuze P, Watelet J, et al. Acute and chronic dissections of the abdominal aorta: clinical features and treatment. J Vasc Surg. 1990;11: 397–402.

Vernhet H, Marty-Ane CH, Lesnik A, et al. Dissection of the abdominal aorta in blunt trauma: management by percutaneous stent placement. Cardiovasc Intervent Radiol. 1997; 20: 473–476.

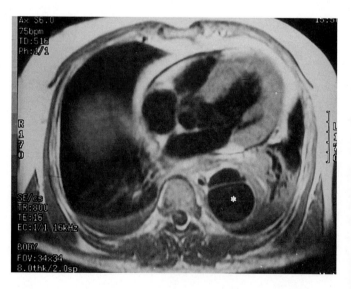

Figure 4–7 Abdominal aortic dissection. T_1-weighted MRI image at the level of the lower thorax. There is an intimal flap separating the anterior true lumen from the posterior false lumen (asterisk). The true lumen is smaller in caliber due to stripping of elastin from its wall.

4.5 UPPER GASTROINTESTINAL BLEEDING

Up to 90% of all gastrointestinal bleeding is from a lesion proximal to the ligament of Treitz, and the most common sites are the gastric body and fundus. The causes of upper gastrointestinal bleeding include peptic ulcer disease, gastrointestinal varices, neoplasms, pancreatitis, hematobilia, and arteriovenous malformations (AVMs). Patients present with hematemesis, melena, and shock. Although endoscopy is the most effective method of diagnosing upper gastrointestinal bleeding, several radiologic examinations (including angiography and nuclear bleeding scans) play a critical role.

Angiography is an alternative when endoscopy fails or is unavailable, and bleeding rates as low as 0.5 mL/min can be detected. Positive angiographic findings include active contrast extravasation and hypervascularity. If a bleeding source is identified on angiography, the vessel responsible may be embolized or treated with intraarterial vasopressin to control the bleeding. Radionuclide bleeding scans using technetium Tc 99m-labeled sulfur colloid and tagged red blood cells (RBCs) are more sensitive than angiography and can detect bleeding rates as low as 0.1 mL/min. Although sulfur colloid studies are easily performed, they are limited by rapid first-pass clearance of tracer by the liver, thus decreasing the chance of identifying intermittent bleeding. Tagged RBC studies are more technically demanding, but they can detect bleeding up to 24 hours after initiation. Scintigraphic findings include an intraluminal focal area of increased activity, or activity that increases with time and that moves through the gastrointestinal tract. Radionuclide studies can be used to triage patients with active bleeding and to localize the approximate bleeding site prior to angiography.

SELECTED REFERENCES

Barth KH. Radiological intervention in upper and lower gastrointestinal bleeding. Baillieres Clin Gastroenterol. 1995; 9: 53–69.

Hamlin JA, Petersen B, Keller FS, Rosch J. Angiographic evaluation and management of nonvariceal upper gastrointestinal bleeding. Gastrointest Endosc Clin North Am. 1997; 7: 703–716.

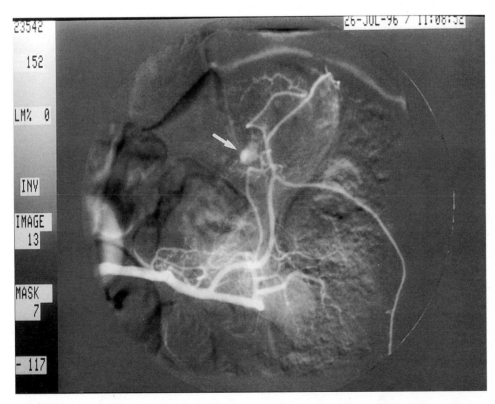

Figure 4–8 Upper GI bleeding. Selective angiography of the short gastric arteries shows extravasation of contrast along the lesser curvature of the stomach (arrow). After multiple failed attempts at endoscopic sclerotherapy, the bleeding was successfully treated by catheter-directed embolization.

4.6 VARICEAL HEMORRHAGE/PORTAL HYPERTENSION

Portal hypertension is defined as elevation of the main portal pressure above 7 mm Hg, and may be classified as presinusoidal, sinusoidal, or postsinusoidal. Presinusoidal causes include extrahepatic portal vein thrombosis or intrahepatic obstruction of the portal venules from a variety of causes, eg, schistosomiasis, hepatic fibrosis, and primary biliary cirrhosis. Postsinusoidal causes are the Budd-Chiari syndrome and hepatic congestion from right-sided heart failure or pericarditis. In the United States, however, the most common cause of portal hypertension occurs at the sinusoidal level from hepatitis or alcohol-related cirrhosis.

Portal hypertension results in the spontaneous formation of multiple portosystemic venous collaterals as an attempt to decompress the portal system. These enlarged venous channels are seen on computed tomography as tubular-enhancing structures within the wall of the esophagus, in the gastrosplenic ligament, in the lesser sac, within the omentum, and along the ligamentum teres (the recanalized umbilical vein). Associated findings on CT, MRI, and ultrasound include ascites, splenomegaly, heterogeneity of the liver, and hepatic nodularity and atrophy with relative sparing of the left lobe and caudate. The diagnosis of a hepatoma, occurring in 4.5% of patients with cirrhosis, is readily seen on cross-sectional imaging.

The major life-threatening emergent complication of portal hypertension is variceal hemorrhage. Esophageal and gastric varices are superficially located beneath the submucosa and are generally well visualized by endoscopy. In addition to the use of somatostatin analogues to diminish splanchnic blood flow, endoscopic ligation or sclerotherapy of varices is often effective for patients who present with bleeding; however, recurrent hemorrhage occurs up to 40% of the time. Arterial portography (delayed imaging after injection of the superior mesenteric artery or splenic artery) or direct portography (by transhepatic puncture or minilaparotomy) allows evaluation of variceal filling and a determination of portal pressure. Percutaneous intrahepatic portosystemic shunting (TIPS) can be performed at the time of angiography, and has proved effective in stopping acute variceal hemorrhage. Any varices that continue to fill after TIPS placement may be occluded by transcatheter embolization techniques, which help to avoid recurrent bleeding. Importantly, in patients without right-sided heart failure, TIPS is associated with a considerably lower morbidity and mortality than emergent surgical portosystemic shunting, and has thus become the technique of choice in patients failing medical or endoscopic therapy.

SELECTED REFERENCES

Kraus BB, Ros PR, Abbitt PL, et al. Comparison of ultrasound, CT and MR imaging in the evaluation of candidates for TIPS. J Magn Reson Imaging. 1995; 5: 571–578.

Komatsuda T, Ishida H, Konno K, et al. Color Doppler findings of gastrointestinal varices. Abdom Imaging. 1998; 23: 45–50.

Johnson CD, Ehman RL, Rakela J, Ilstrup DM. MR angiography in portal hypertension: detection of varices and imaging techniques. J Comput Assist Tomogr. 1991; 15: 578–584.

Rossle M, Siegerstetter V, Huber M, Ochs A. The first decade of the transjugular intrahepatic portosystemic shunt (TIPS): state of the art. Liver. 1998; 18: 73–89.

Kerlan RK, LaBerge JM, Gordon RL, Ring EJ. Transjugular intrahepatic portosystemic shunts: current status. AJR. 1995; 164: 1059–1066.

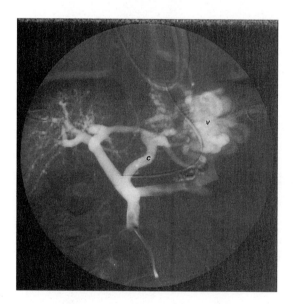
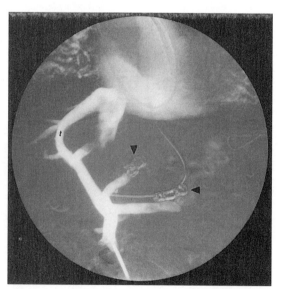

Figure 4–9 Variceal hemorrhage. Direct transmesenteric portography (**left**) revealing enlargement of the coronary (**c**) and short gastric veins supplying multiple retrogastric and esophageal varices (**v**). After transvenous intrahepatic portosystemic shunt placement (**right**) and coil embolization of the coronary and gastric veins (arrowheads), the varices are almost completely occluded (**T** marks the TIPS shunt).

4.7 LOWER GASTROINTESTINAL BLEEDING

Lower gastrointestinal (LGI) bleeding, defined as bleeding from a source distal to the ligament of Treitz, accounts for 10–15% of intestinal hemorrhage. The most common cause is diverticulosis, although other potential colonic causes include inflammatory bowel disease, ischemic and infectious colitis, arteriovenous malformations (AVMs), and tumors. Small bowel bleeding from AVMs, diverticuli, or neoplastic disease is responsible for approximately 3–5% of LGI bleeding. An aortoenteric fistula is a potentially catastrophic event and should always be considered when evaluating patients with abdominal aortic aneurysms or previous aortic surgery.

Colonoscopy successfully identifies the bleeding source in most cases, and may permit appropriate endoscopic therapy. Radionuclide scanning using Tc 99m tagged red blood cells or sulfur colloid may be used to diagnose active intermittent bleeding, and has a sensitivity of 0.1 to 0.5 mL/min. Selective mesenteric angiography is reserved for patients who are unable to undergo colonoscopy or who fail endoscopic management. Angiographic determination of the bleeding source is possible in approximately one half of cases, and findings include contrast extravasation, arteriovenous shunting, and hyperemia. When bleeding is identified, the transcatheter infusion of vasopressin or catheter-directed superselective vascular occlusion (embolization) successfully stops bleeding in most cases. Should these measures fail, surgical resection of the affected segment of bowel is associated with low morbidity and high rates of success.

SELECTED REFERENCES

Vernava AM, Moore BA, Longo WE, Johnson FE. Lower gastrointestinal bleeding. Dis Colon Rectum. 1997; 40: 846–858.

Manten HD, Green JA. Acute lower gastrointestinal bleeding. A guide to initial management. Postgrad Med. 1995; 97: 154–157.

Gordon RL, Ahl KL, Kerlan RK, et al. Selective arterial embolization for the control of lower gastrointestinal bleeding. Am J Surg. 1997; 174: 24–28.

Guy GE, Shetty PC, Sharma RP, et al. Acute lower gastrointestinal hemorrhage: treatment by superselective embolization with polyvinyl alcohol particles. AJR. 1992; 159: 521–526.

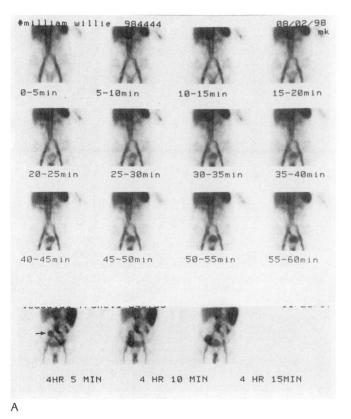

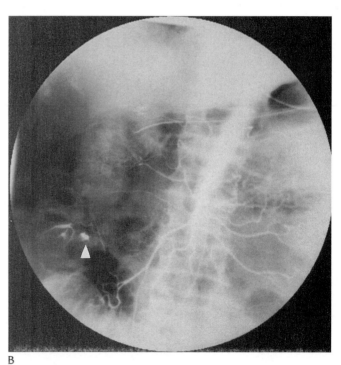

A   B

Figure 4–10A, B Lower GI bleeding. Nuclear bleeding scan using Tc 99m-labeled red blood cells (**A**). On delayed imaging there is increased activity seen in the right lower quadrant of the abdomen (4 h 5 min), representing radiotracer extravasation into the bowel lumen (arrow). A corresponding selective superior mesenteric arteriogram (**B**) on the same patient shows active bleeding from a colonic diverticulum (arrowhead).

4.8 ACUTE INTESTINAL ISCHEMIA

Acute mesenteric ischemia (MI) may be from occlusive and nonocclusive causes. The origin of occlusive MI in 50% of the cases is embolic obstruction of the superior mesenteric artery alone, and emboli to multiple vessels is responsible for another 20% of cases. The most common source of emboli are cardiac (eg, in patients with atrial fibrillation), although other sources include aortic aneurysms and atheromatous plaque. Clinically, patients present with severe, colicky abdominal pain. Physical findings are surprisingly benign unless bowel infarction and peritonitis has occurred. Early angiography is necessary to diagnose embolic occlusion before the onset of bowel necrosis. Findings include an abrupt vessel "cutoff," intraluminal filling defects at the vessel origin or arterial branch points, and stasis of contrast. Embolic occlusion of the superior mesenteric artery is a surgical emergency owing to poor prognosis if intestinal necrosis ensues. Nonoccluding thromboemboli can be treated with anticoagulation and thrombolytic therapy.

Nonocclusive mesenteric ischemia represents a low flow state and is primarily a disease of elderly patients with coexistent cardiac disease. Intestinal ischemia is caused by severe vasoconstriction of the mesenteric vascular bed occurring as a response to shock, hypovolemia, decreased cardiac output, or medications (ergot alkaloids, digitalis). Vasoconstriction can persist after correction of the precipitating event, and in these patients emergent angiography is indicated. Angiographic findings include extreme vasoconstriction of the mesenteric vascular bed, diminished mucosal enhancement, poor venous opacification, and reflux of contrast back into the aorta. Once diagnosed, treatment can be started immediately with the transcatheter intraarterial infusion of the vasodilator papavarine directly into the superior mesenteric artery.

There are no reliable plain film findings of intestinal ischemia. When air is seen in the bowel wall, intestinal infarction has already occurred. CT can detect ischemic bowel, which appears as thickened, dilated, and fluid-filled loops of bowel. Barium studies show lumen narrowing with "thumbprinting" or the "stack of coins" sign. Physiologically, these phenomena are caused by bowel wall edema and hemorrhage.

SELECTED REFERENCES

Schutz A, Eichinger W, Breuer M, et al. Acute mesenteric ischemia: diagnosis with contrast-enhanced CT. Radiology. 1996; 49: 632–636.

Lock G, Scholmerich J. Non-occlusive mesenteric ischemia. Hepatogastroenterology. 1995; 42: 234–239.

Kaleya RN, Sammartano RJ, Boley SJ. Aggressive approach to acute mesenteric ischemia. Surg Clin North Am. 1992; 72: 157–182.

Figure 4–11 Acute occlusive mesenteric ischemia. Acute mesenteric ischemia due to embolic occlusion of the superior mesenteric artery (SMA) in a patient with known atrial fibrillation. Abrupt cutoff of the SMA is noted (arrow).

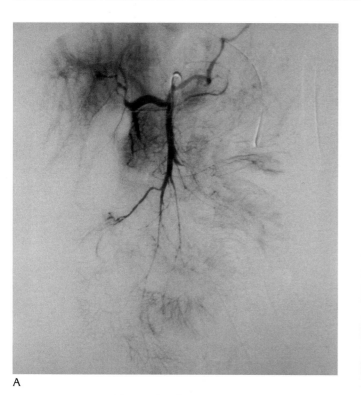

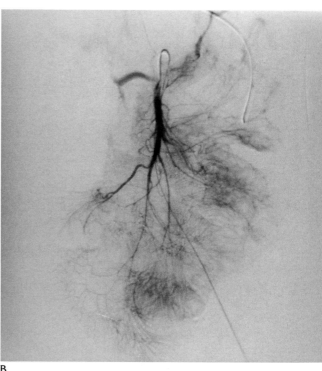

A   B

Figure 4–12A, B Nonocclusive mesenteric ischemia in a patient taking digitalis.
Selective angiography of the superior mesenteric artery (**A**) reveals marked vasoconstriction and diminished mucosal enhancement. After an overnight infusion of papaverine, there is decreased spasm and improved mucosal perfusion (**B**).

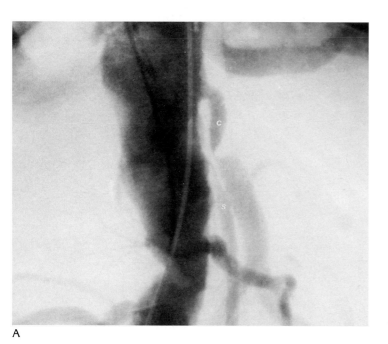

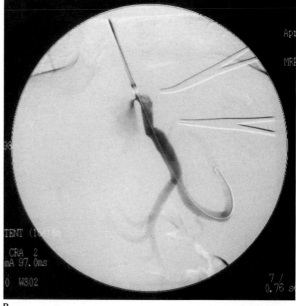

A   B

Figure 4–13A, B Chronic mesenteric ischemia. A lateral abdominal aortogram (**A**) shows marked atherosclerotic narrowing of the celiac trunk (**c**) and the superior mesenteric artery (SMA) (**s**). After percutaneous angioplasty and stent placement, the celiac is widely patent (**B**). A stent was also successfully placed in the SMA.

4.9 ATHEROMATOUS RENAL ARTERY STENOSIS

Renal artery stenosis (RAS) occurs in up to 5% of patients with hypertension, and is increasingly recognized as a cause of renal dysfunction. Atherosclerosis is responsible for 60–75% of cases of RAS, and bilateral involvement occurs in 33% of patients. Three quarters of lesions are ostial, and are primarily the result of aortic plaques that overhang and compromise the renal artery orifice. Atheromatous plaques occur less commonly in the distal renal artery and its branches. Untreated, the natural history of atheromatous RAS is progressive stenosis and occlusion, with associated renal atrophy and functional impairment.

Although angiography is at present the reference standard for evaluating atherosclerotic RAS, several other imaging modalities have gained widespread acceptance for the evaluation of the renal vasculature. Principal among these is renal duplex sonography (RDS), which has a reported sensitivity of 95% and specificity of 90% for detecting a stenosis of ≥60%. The basis for the diagnosis of RAS is Doppler determinations of blood flow rather than imaging of the actual stenosis. Peak systolic velocities of >180 cm/sec in the main renal artery and alterations in the spectral pattern of intrarenal arteries are diagnostic. The usefulness of RDS is limited by operator and site experience, poor imaging of patients with tortuous renal anatomy or a large body habitus, and an inability to reliably demonstrate multiple or accessory renal arteries.

Three-dimensional gadolinium-enhanced magnetic resonance angiography (MRA) can provide images similar to arteriograms for evaluating renal artery stenosis. Limitations include a difficulty in evaluating branch vessels and accessory arteries, patient motion, and metal artifacts. In addition, MRA techniques tend to overestimate the severity of lesions.

CTA can also provide images similar to arteriograms, but CTA requires large doses of contrast and is also limited in its ability to evaluate small accessory vessels. Concomitant aortic and visceral vessel evaluation makes CTA an attractive modality because these patients universally have diffuse disease.

Captopril-stimulated nuclear studies image renal function and indirectly assess renal blood flow. Renal artery stenosis is implied by decreased and delayed renal uptake or washout of the radiolabeled tracer after the administration of captopril. This test has a 90% sensitivity and 95% specificity for renal artery stenosis, but is less reliable in patients with impaired renal function.

SELECTED REFERENCES

Zierler RE, Bergelin RO, Davidson RC, et al. A prospective study of disease progression in patients with atherosclerotic renal artery disease. Am J Hypertens. 1996; 9: 1055–1061.

Mittal BR, Kumar P, Arora P, et al. Role of captopril renography in the diagnosis of renovascular hypertension. Am J Kid Dis. 1996; 28: 209–213.

Stavros T, Harshfield D. Renal doppler, renal artery stenosis, and renovascular hypertension:direct and indirect sonographic abnormalities in patients with renal artery stenosis. Ultrasound Q 1994; 12: 217–263.

Losinno F, Zuccala A, Busato F, Zucchelli P. Renal artery angioplasty for renovascular hypertension and preservation of renal function: long-term angiographic and clinical follow-up. AJR. 1994; 162: 853–857.

Rundback JH, Gray R, Rozenblit G, et al. Renal artery stent placement for the management of ischemic nephropathy. J Vasc Intervent Radiol. 1997; 8: 40–45.

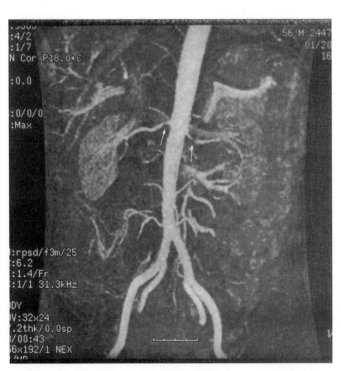

Figure 4–14 Atheromatous renal artery stenosis. Coronal gradient-echo MRI shows bilateral proximal renal artery stenosis (arrows). Mild poststenotic dilatation is also seen on both sides.

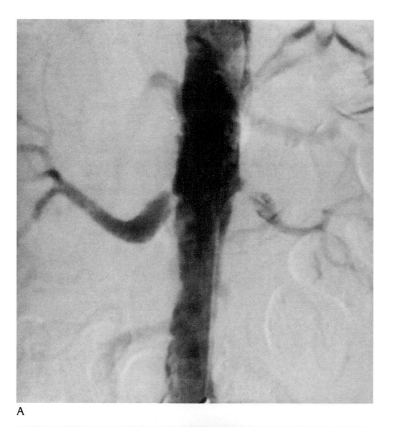

A

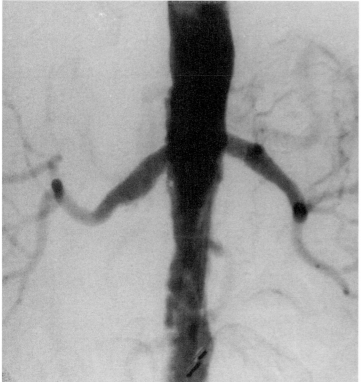

B

Figure 4–15A, B Atheromatous renal artery stenosis. An abdominal aortogram (**A**) reveals severe ostial narrowing of the renal arteries bilaterally. Note the extensive atherosclerotic irregularity of the aorta. After bilateral renal angioplasty and stent placement, the caliber of both renal arteries is normal (**B**).

4.10 RENAL ARTERY FIBROMUSCULAR DYSPLASIA

Fibromuscular dysplasia (FMD) accounts for roughly one third of cases of renal artery stenosis. Although there are several histologic variants, approximately 85% are the result of medial fibroplasia. The pathogenesis of this condition is uncertain. FMD is manifested clinically by the development of hypertension in women during their 3rd and 4th decades of life. The disease is rare in blacks. Although renal duplex sonography or radionuclide renal scans may identify the presence of a hemodynamically significant lesion, angiography is necessary both to characterize the lesion and provide definitive treatment. Angiographically, medial fibroplasia has a characteristic "string-of-beads" appearance because of alternating areas of weblike stenosis and poststenotic dilatation. Lesions are usually nonostial within the main renal artery, but may involve branch vessels in approximately 20% of cases. The disease is bilateral in two thirds of patients. Although progressive arterial occlusion

and associated renal atrophy is uncommon, potential complications include spontaneous dissection, aneurysm formation, and renal infarcts. Percutaneous transluminal angioplasty is successful in correcting the renal artery stenosis and curing or improving hypertension in more than 90% of patients.

SELECTED REFERENCES

Pohl MA, Novick AC. Natural history of atherosclerotic and fibrous renal artery disease: clinical implications. Am J Kid Dis. 1985; 5: A120–130.

Tegtmeyer CJ, Selby JB, Hartwell GD, et al. Results and complications of angioplasty in fibromuscular disease. Circulation. 1991; 83(suppl 2): II155–161.

Cicuto KP, McLean GK, Oleaga JA, et al. Renal artery stenosis: anatomic classification for percutaneous transluminal angioplasty. AJR. 1981; 137: 599–601.

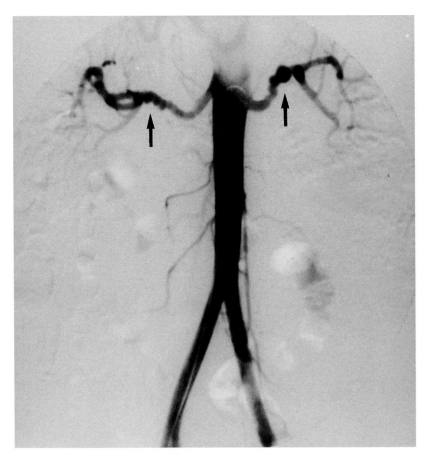

Figure 4–16 Fibromuscular dysplasia of the renal arteries. Abdominal aortography shows "beading" of both main renal arteries caused by medial fibroplasia (arrows). This was subsequently treated by balloon angioplasty.

4.11 ACUTE CHOLECYSTITIS

Acute cholecystitis is associated with gallstones in 95% of patients, and approximately one third of patients with gallstones develop acute cholecystitis. The pathogenesis is stone impaction in the gallbladder neck or cystic duct, causing inflammation and patchy necrosis of the gallbladder wall. Women are affected three times more commonly than men. Patients commonly present with right upper quadrant abdominal pain, and the differential diagnosis includes pancreatitis, peptic ulcer disease, hepatitis, appendicitis, and perihepatitis (Fitz-Hugh-Curtis syndrome). Acalculous cholecystitis may occur following total parenteral nutrition, anesthesia, sepsis and shock, surgery, and infectious causes.

Sonography is the modality of choice to confirm the diagnosis of acute cholecystitis. The most sensitive criterion for diagnosing acute cholecystitis is the presence of a sonographic Murphy's sign, which is maximal tenderness over the gallbladder, in association with gallstones. Other sonographic signs are gallbladder sludge, gallbladder dilatation, wall thickening (>3 mm) with intramural sonolucency, and pericholecystic fluid.

Cholescintigraphy should be used to diagnose acute cholecystitis if ultrasonography is equivocal. The diagnosis is made when the gallbladder is not visualized within 60 minutes of being injected with technetium 99m disofenin. The "rim sign," an arc-shaped area of increased activity in the gallbladder fossa following hyperemia, is seen in approximately 25% of patients with acute cholecystitis. Patients need to fast for 4 hours before the procedure; prolonged fasting (>24 hours) and hepatic insufficiency may result in false-positive examinations.

SELECTED REFERENCES

Vasilescu C, Jovin GH, Popescu I, Esanu C. Decision analysis in the clinical and imaging diagnosis of acute cholecystitis. Med Interne. 1990; 14: 329–340.

Zeman RK, Garra BS. Gallbladder imaging. The state of the art. Gastroenterol Clin North Am. 1991; 14: 127–156.

Babb RR. Acute acalculous cholecystitis. A review. J Clin Gastroenterol. 1992; 14: 238–241.

Loud PA, Semelka RC, Kettritz U, et al. MRI of acute cholecystitis: comparison with the normal gallbladder and other entities. Magn Reson Imaging. 1996; 14: 349–355.

Schiller VL, Turner RR, Sarti DA. Color doppler imaging of the gallbladder wall in acute cholecystitis: sonographic-pathologic correlation. Abdom Imaging. 1996; 32: 233–237.

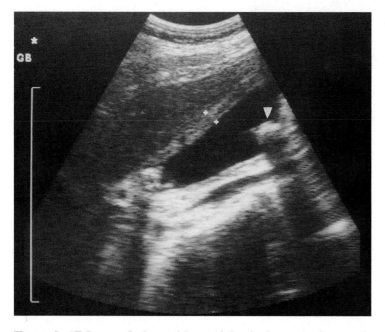

Figure 4–17 Acute cholecystitis. Abdominal sonography reveals thickening of the gallbladder wall with intramural edema (cursors) and a gallstone with associated acoustical shadowing is visualized. A sonographic Murphy's sign was also present.

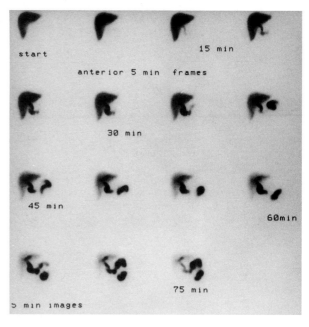

Figure 4–18 Acute cholecystitis. A hepatobiliary scan shows uptake of radioisotope within the liver and excretion into the small bowel. There is nonvisualization of the gallbladder.

4.12 CHRONIC CHOLECYSTITIS

Chronic cholecystitis is caused by transient obstruction of the gallbladder neck or cystic duct by a gallstone. Patients usually complain of recurrent colicky right upper quadrant pain that lasts for several hours. The basis of the diagnosis is clinical findings, and these can be confirmed by sonographic demonstration of gallbladder wall thickening that cannot be attributed to nonbiliary causes. Nuclear studies are usually normal in patients with chronic cholecystitis, although delayed visualization of the gallbladder (5%) or delayed biliary-to-bowel transit time are occasionally seen. Determination of a reduced gallbladder ejection fraction (30%) after the administration of cholecystokinin is also associated with chronic cholecystitis and biliary dyskinesia.

SELECTED REFERENCES

Goldberg HI. Imaging of the biliary tract. Curr Opin Radiol. 1992; 14: 62–69.

Goldberg HI, Gordon R. Diagnostic and interventional procedures for the biliary tract. Curr Opin Radiol. 1991; 3: 453–462.

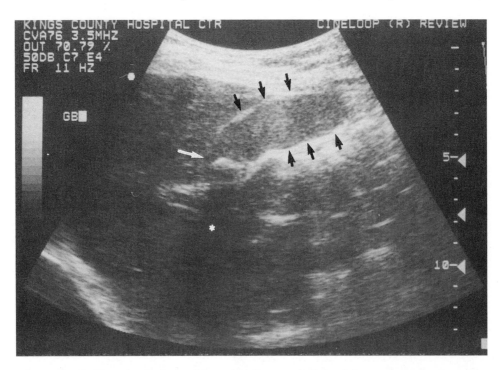

Figure 4–19 Chronic cholecystitis.   An ultrasound of the right upper quadrant reveals a distended, sludge-filled gallbladder (arrows), causing the gallbladder to appear echogenic. A stone is noted at the neck of the gallbladder (white arrow), resulting in posterior acoustical shadowing (asterisk).

4.13 EMPHYSEMATOUS CHOLECYSTITIS

Emphysematous cholecystitis is a rare form of acute cholecystitis in which the gallbladder is infected with a gas-forming organism. It differs from the usual type of cholecystitis in that stones are usually absent; men are more commonly affected than women, 38% of patients are diabetic, and gangrene of the gallbladder with resulting perforation is 5 times more common.

There is an increased prevalence in patients with diabetes. Although traditionally considered a surgical emergency, percutaneous drainage (cholecystostomy) may be used in selected high-risk patients. Emphysematous cholecystitis has a characteristic appearance on sonography, with multiple hyperechoic foci representing gas bubbles. If intramural, these foci take an arc-like configuration. If intraluminal, the hyperechoic foci are nondependent and an associated "ring down" artifact is usually present. CT is highly sensitive for the detection of abnormal gas collections, and should be performed to confirm the diagnosis. Gas may also be seen on abdominal plain films, but radiography is much less sensitive.

SELECTED REFERENCES

Gill KS, Chapman AH, Weston MJ. The changing face of emphysematous cholecystitis. Br J Radiol. 1997; 70: 986–991.

Vingan HL, Wohlgemuth SD, Bell JS. Percutaneous cholecystostomy drainage for the treatment of acute emphysematous cholecystitis. AJR. 1990; 155: 1013–1014.

Lee BY, Morilla CV. Acute emphysematous cholecystitis: a case report and review of the literature. NY State J Med. 1992; 92: 406–407.

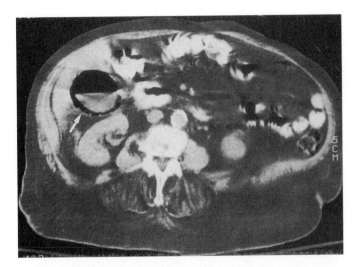

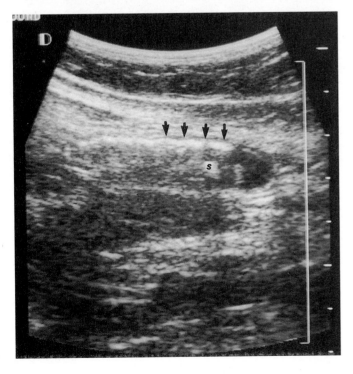

Figure 4–20 Emphysematous cholecystitis. Air is seen in the wall of the gallbladder on CT (arrow).

Figure 4–21 Emphysematous cholecystitis. An abdominal ultrasound shows increased echogenicity in the gallbladder wall due to intramural air (arrows). A stone is also noted (**s**).

4.14 PYELONEPHRITIS

Acute pyelonephritis usually results from an ascending urinary tract infection, and females between the ages of 15 and 35 years are most frequently infected. Gram-negative organisms are responsible for >85% of cases. The disease is usually unilateral, but may be bilateral. Diabetes is an important predisposing medical condition. Radiographic imaging, including sonography and CT, is usually reserved for patients who do not respond to appropriate antibiotic therapy, to rule out obstruction or abscess formation.

Uncomplicated acute pyelonephritis usually does not display any abnormality on sonography. Occasionally, renal enlargement with areas of decreased echogenicity representing edema may be seen. Contrast-enhanced CT reveals an enlarged kidney with focal areas of decreased attenuation. Progression to

emphysematous pyelonephritis, a necrotizing process, is rare. In such cases, air in the parenchyma and collecting system may be evident on CT or ultrasound.

SELECTED REFERENCES

Kawashima A, Sandler CM, Goldman SM. Current roles and controversies in the imaging evaluation of acute renal infection. World J Urol. 1998; 16: 9–17.

Kaplan DM, Rosenfield AT, Smith RC. Advances in the imaging of renal infection. Helical CT and modern coordinated imaging. Infect Dis Clin North Am. 1997; 11: 681–705.

Bailey RR, Lynn KL, Robson RA, et al. DMSA renal scans in adults with acute pyelonephritis. Clin Nephrol. 1996; 46: 99–104.

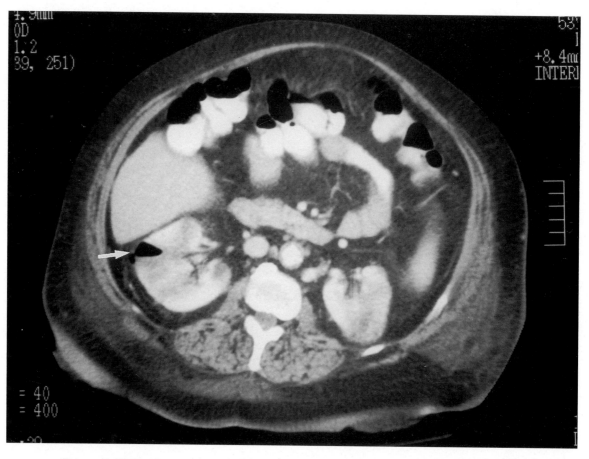

Figure 4–22 Emphysematous pyelonephritis. A contrast-enhanced CT scan through the mid-abdomen shows a focal collection of air within the right kidney (arrow).

4.15 APPENDICITIS

Acute appendicitis is caused by obstruction of the lumen of the appendix, and results in right lower quadrant abdominal pain, fever, nausea and vomiting, and leukocytosis. Localized tenderness is generally present over the inflamed appendix. Plain films of the abdomen may show a paucity of bowel gas in the right lower quadrant of the abdomen, loss of the psoas margin and properitoneal fat pad, and thickening of the wall of the cecum. A laminated calcified appendicolith is present in approximately 10% of cases, and is more common in children. The diagnosis is confirmed using ultrasound or computed tomography (CT). Ultrasound is accurate in almost 95% of cases, and shows a thickened, distended, noncompressible aperistaltic tubular structure representing the inflamed appendix. Localized periappendiceal fluid may be present, although large amounts of intraperitoneal fluid are suggestive of appendiceal rupture. CT is highly sensitive in revealing the dilated and thick-walled appendix and surrounding inflammatory changes. In addition, complications such as rupture or abscess formation are well demonstrated. Treatment is open surgical or laparoscopic appendectomy.

SELECTED REFERENCES

Incesu L, Coskun A, Selcuk MB, et al. Acute appendicitis: MR imaging and sonographic correlation. AJR. 1997; 168: 669–674.

Curtin KR, Fitzgerald SW, Nemcek AA, et al. CT diagnosis of acute appendicitis: imaging findings. AJR. 1995; 164: 905–909.

Gupta H, Dupuy DE. Advances in imaging of the acute abdomen. Surg Clin North Am. 1997; 168: 1245–1263.

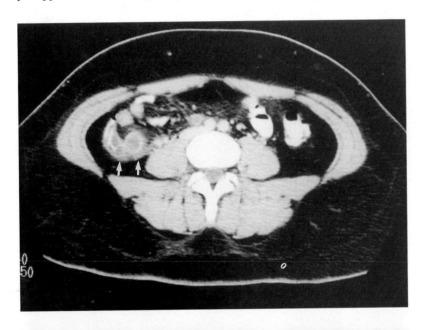

Figure 4–23 Appendicitis. A CT scan shows the appendix as dilated and fluid filled (arrows). The adjacent mesenteric fat shows inflammatory changes.

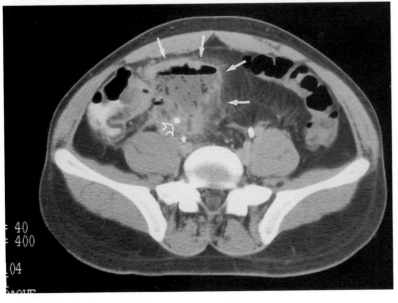

Figure 4–24 Appendiceal abscess. A CT of the pelvis reveals thickening of the appendix and an adjacent collection (arrows) containing air-fluid levels. An appendicolith (open arrow) is identified within the dependent portion of the abscess. The contrast-opacified ureters are in their normal location on the anterior aspect of the psoas muscles.

4.16 CROHN'S DISEASE

Crohn's disease is a chronic transmural inflammatory process of uncertain origin. Distal small bowel and colonic involvement are the most common presentation, and represent 45% of cases. Small bowel involvement alone is seen in 30% of cases and the remaining 25% of cases involve solely the colon.

The radiologic evaluation of Crohn's disease begins with an abdominal plain film, which may show thickened folds and an abnormal gas pattern. A double-contrast barium study is often diagnostic, and characteristic findings include apthous ulcers, a "cobblestone" appearance of the bowel, fistulas, "skip lesions," and strictures. CT and MRI are extremely helpful in evaluating associated abdominal complications such as abscess formation. Other CT findings include bowel wall thickening ("donut sign"), "creeping fat" (progressive increase in mesenteric fat over the inflamed serosal surface), and intra-abdominal phlegmons. There is a slight increase in small bowel malignancies in patients with Crohn's disease.

Nuclear studies using indium In 111-labeled leukocytes may be useful in assessing disease progression or response to ther-apy. Percutaneous image-guided drainage is an effective palliative procedure in patients with associated intra-abdominal abscesses.

SELECTED REFERENCES

Ernst O, Asselah T, Cablan X, Sergent G. Breath-hold fast spin-echo MR imaging of Crohn's disease. AJR. 1998; 170: 127–128.

Haggett PJ, Moore NR, Shearman JD, et al. Pelvic and perineal complications of Crohn's disease: assessment using magnetic resonance imaging. Gut. 1995; 36: 407–410.

Sarrazin J, Wilson SR. Manifestation of Crohn disease at US. Radiographics. 1996; 16: 499–520.

Navab F, Boyd CM. Clinical utility of In-111 leukocyte imaging of Crohn's disease. Clin Nucl Med. 1995; 20: 1065–1069.

Sahai A, Belair M, Gianfelice D, et al. Percutaneous drainage of intra-abdominal abscesses in Crohn's disease: short and long-term outcome. Am J Gastroenterol. 1997; 92: 275–278.

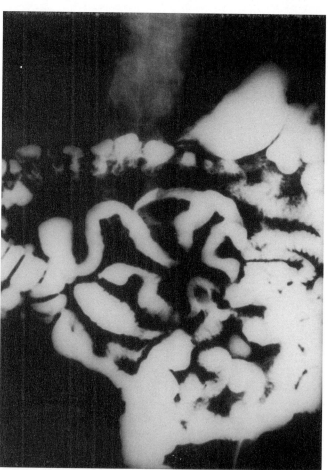

A

B

Figure 4–25A, B Crohn's disease. Upper GI series shows wall thickening, loss of mucosal markings, and separation of small bowel loops (**A**). A CT scan (**B**) of the same patient better reveals the thickening of the bowel wall.

4.17 PSEUDOMEMBRANOUS COLITIS

Pseudomembranous colitis occurs most commonly as a complication of antibiotic therapy, although immunodeficiency and chronic debilitating diseases may also be predisposing factors. *Clostridium difficile* overgrowth is implicated in the pathogenesis, and histology of affected patients reveals fibrinous pseudomembranes covering areas of denuded colonic mucosa. Radiographs of the abdomen often show dilatation of the colon with "thumbprinting" due to haustral thickening. Scintigraphic imaging with In 111-labeled leukocytes will show colonic localization. CT shows a homogeneously enhancing and thickened colonic wall; pericolonic inflammation may also be noted. Imaging findings of air in the colonic wall (pneumatosis coli) or progressive dilatation of the colon in a systemically toxic patient may forebode the development of toxic megacolon, and represents a surgical emergency. Treatment consists of par-enteral vancomycin and discontinuation of the offending antibiotic.

SELECTED REFERENCES

Johnson GL, Johnson PT, Fishman EK. CT evaluation of the acute abdomen: bowel pathology spectrum of disease. Crit Rev Diagn Imaging. 1996; 20: 163–190.

Hamrick KM, Tishler JM, Schwartz ML, et al. The CT findings in pseudomembranous colitis. Comput Med Imaging Graph. 1989; 13: 343–346.

Nathan MA, Seabold JE, Brown BP, Bushnell DL. Colonic localization of labeled leukocytes in critically ill patients. Scintigraphic detection of pseudomembranous colitis. Clin Nucl Med. 1995; 20: 99–106.

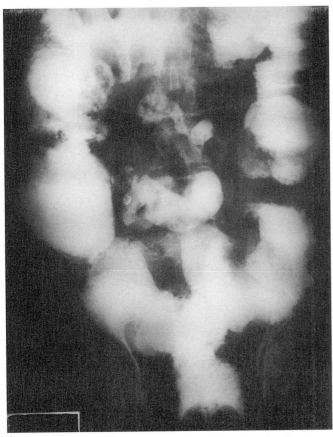

A

B

Figure 4–26A, B Pseudomembranous colitis. A barium enema (**A**) reveals dilatation of the colon with loss of haustration, intramural edema ("thumbprinting"), and internal debris due to the pseudomembranes. On CT (**B**), there is marked circumferential edema of the colon wall (arrows).

4.18 DIVERTICULITIS

Diverticulosis is a disease of industrialized nations that was relatively uncommon before this century. Diverticuli are saclike outpouchings of mucosa and submucosa that extend through the colonic wall. The term diverticulosis refers to the presence of asymptomatic diverticuli, whereas symptomatic patients with diverticular inflammation or other complications are said to have diverticulitis. Today, 60–70% of patients 60 years of age or older who are examined by barium enema will have diverticuli. Their origin is believed to be the result of increased colonic transit time and abnormally high intracolonic luminal pressure. Diverticuli occur at the site of penetrating blood vessels, where there is natural wall weakness. Their close anatomical association with blood vessels accounts for a high incidence of hemorrhage. Although diverticuli occur most commonly in the sigmoid colon, bleeding diverticuli are more often found in the right colon. Patients with diverticulosis can be asymptomatic, or they can present with cramping, altered bowel habits, or lower gastrointestinal bleeding. In fact, diverticular disease is the most common cause of colonic bleeding in adults.

Diverticulitis develops when a diverticulum becomes occluded, resulting in microperforations and inflammatory changes. This can progress to frank intra-abdominal abscesses and colonic strictures. Unlike diverticulosis, diverticulitis almost never is associated with colonic bleeding. CT is an excellent modality for diagnosing diverticular disease and its complications. Small air bubbles can be seen adjacent to the bowel wall representing air in the diverticuli. Oral or colonic contrast can also be seen as small collections adjacent to the bowel wall. Infiltration of the mesenteric and pericolic fat as well as thickened edematous bowel are typical findings seen with diverticulitis. Associated abscesses can also be seen. Although not the procedure of choice, a barium enema is also helpful in diagnosing diverticulitis, demonstrating colonic narrowing and spasm, mass effect, fistulas, and barium in diverticuli.

SELECTED REFERENCES

Rao PM, Rhea JT, Novelline RA, et al. Helical CT with only colonic contrast material for diagnosing diverticulitis: prospective evaluation of 150 patients. AJR. 1998; 170: 1445–1449.

Jacobs JE, Birnbaum BA. CT of inflammatory disease of the colon. Semin Ultrasound CT MR. 1995; 16: 91–101.

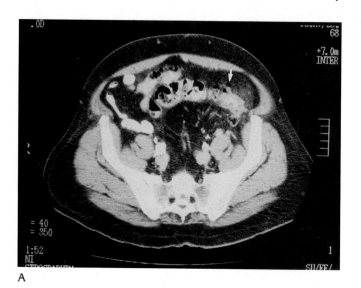 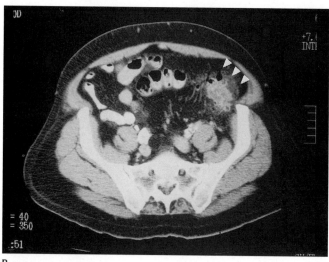

A B

Figure 4–27A, B Diverticulitis. A pelvic CT illustrates focal thickening of the sigmoid colon (**A**). Air seen adjacent to the bowel is within a diverticulum (arrow). A slightly more caudal image (**B**) shows inflammatory changes within the mesentery (arrowheads).

4.19 PANCREATITIS

Acute pancreatitis most often occurs as a result of alcohol ingestion or gallstone disease. Other causes include trauma, infections, certain drugs, and metabolic disorders. Clinically, patients present with abdominal pain that radiates to the back. Amylase and lipase levels in the blood are elevated and calcium levels are often found to be reduced.

Acute pancreatitis causes enlargement of part of or the entire pancreas due to inflammation and edema. CT is the radiologic procedure of choice for diagnosing pancreatitis and is a useful prognosticator of patient outcome. On CT, the pancreas is enlarged and there is usually decreased parenchymal attenuation as a result of edema. Nonenhancing areas represent foci of pancreatic necrosis. Inflammatory infiltration of the peripancreatic fat and peripancreatic fluid collections are well seen. The treatment of choice is surgical debridement and partial pancreatectomy, although focal fluid collections and small areas of pancreatic necrosis may be drained percutaneously.

Sonography usually reveals a large pancreas, which is hypoechoic and has a poorly defined contour. Ultrasound is often limited in these patients because of the severity of the patients' abdominal tenderness as well as increased overlying bowel gas caused by a frequently associated ileus. MRI may be used to show the extent of pancreatic inflammation and local complications, and has the advantage of not requiring the intravenous administration of iodine-containing contrast material.

SELECTED REFERENCES

De Sanctis JT, Lee MJ, Gazelle GS, et al. Prognostic indicators in acute pancreatitis: CT vs APACHE II. Clin Radiol. 1997; 52: 842–848.

Morgan DE, Baron TH, Smith JK, et al. Pancreatic fluid collections prior to intervention: evaluation with MR imaging compared with CT and US. Radiology. 1997; 203: 773–778.

Echenique AM, Sleeman D, Yrizarry J, et al. Percutaneous catheter-directed debridement of infected pancreatic necrosis: results in 20 patients. J Vasc Interv Radiol. 1998; 9: 565–571.

Balthazar EJ, Robinson DL, Megibow AJ, Ranson JH. Acute pancreatitis: value of CT in establishing prognosis. Radiology. 1990; 174: 331–336.

Feig BW, Pomerantz RA, Vogelzang R, et al. Treatment of peripancreatic fluid collections in patients with complicated acute pancreatitis. Surg Gynecol Obstet. 1992; 52: 429–436.

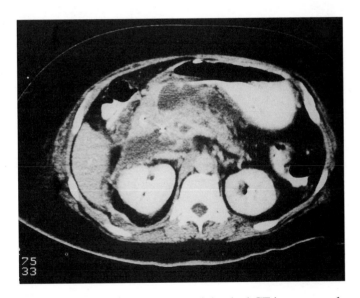

Figure 4–28 Pancreatitis. An abdominal CT image reveals pancreatic necrosis with an extensive associated retroperitoneal phlegmon.

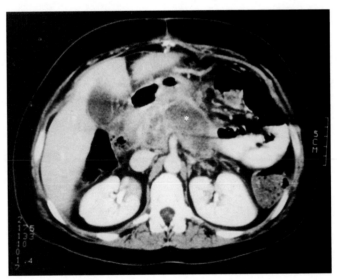

Figure 4–29 Pancreatitis. CT scan on a different patient shows a well-organized collection in the pancreatic bed, consistent with a pseudocyst (asterisk).

4.20 INTRA-ABDOMINAL ABSCESS

Intra-abdominal abscesses represent infected fluid collections that develop after surgery or as a result of inflammatory intra-abdominal conditions (eg, diverticulitis, pancreatitis, appendicitis, inflammatory bowel disease). Collections tend to develop adjacent to the inflammatory process but may spread with the aid of gravity to involve adjacent peritoneal recesses. Untreated, intra-abdominal abscesses result in hematogenous bacterial seeding and sepsis and an associated mortality approaching 30%. Early recognition and appropriate management can have a major impact on patient outcome. Nuclear medicine techniques allow identification of inflammatory foci, and can differentiate infected from benign fluid collections. However, computed tomography and ultrasonography are the principal imaging tools used to diagnose abdominal fluid collections and their underlying cause. Image-guided aspiration and drainage is used for both diagnostic and therapeutic purposes, and percutaneous drainage is associated with clinical success in most cases. Surgical debridement is reserved for interloop abscesses, multiloculated collections, abscesses with large enteric fistula, inaccessible abscesses, infected hematomas that fail to drain after the intracavitary administration of thrombolytic agents, and abscesses that fail percutaneous therapy.

SELECTED REFERENCES

Datz FL. Abdominal abscess detection: gallium, [111]In-, and ^{99m}Tc-labeled leukocytes, and polyclonal and monoclonal antibodies. Semin Nucl Med. 1996; 26: 51–64.

Adam EJ, Page JE. Intra-abdominal sepsis: the role of radiology. Baillieres Clin Gastroenterol. 1991; 5 (3 Pt 1): 587–609.

Montgomery RS, Wilson SE. Intraabdominal abscesses: image-guided diagnosis and therapy. Clin Infect Dis. 1996; 23: 28–36.

DeMeo JH, Fulcher AS, Austin RF Jr. Anatomic CT demonstration of the peritoneal spaces, ligaments, and mesenteries: normal and pathologic processes. Radiographics. 1995; 15: 755–770.

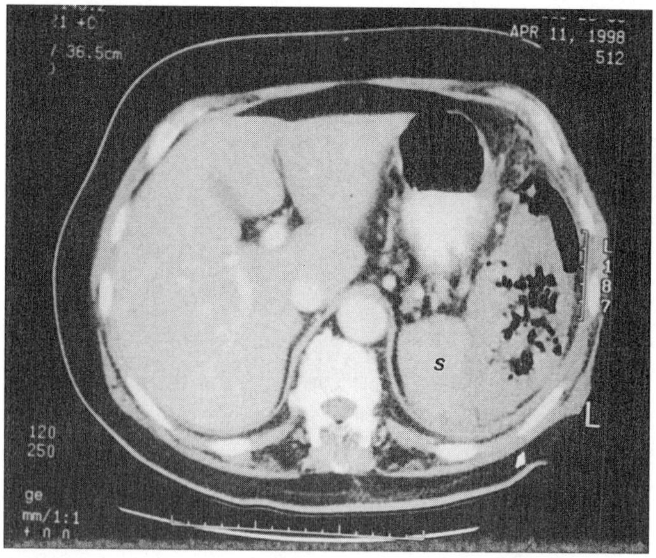

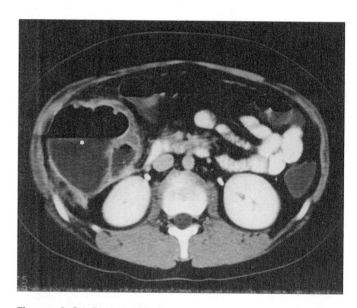

Figure 4–30 Intra-abdominal abscess. A CT image of the upper abdomen reveals a collection that contains multiple air bubbles adjacent to the spleen (**s**).

Figure 4–31 Intra-abdominal abscess. A large air-fluid collection is noted in the right lower quadrant (asterisk). There is infiltration of the adjacent fat.

4.21 PELVIC INFLAMMATORY DISEASE/TUBO-OVARIAN ABSCESS

Pelvic inflammatory disease (PID) affects 8 million women annually in the United States. Chlamydia is the most common pathogen; gonorrhea occurs less frequently. Patients usually present with pain, cervical motion tenderness, a purulent discharge, and fever. Approximately 25% of women will experience long-term complications including infertility and ectopic pregnancy. As the disease process becomes more severe, an abscess can develop. Ultrasound is the modality of choice when evaluating patients with suspected PID.

Ultrasound findings depend on the severity of the disease. Early disease may only show an enlargement of the adnexa with loss of tissue planes. As the disease progresses, ill-defined hypoechoic areas may be seen, and there can be associated free fluid in the pelvic cul-de-sac. Late in the course of the disease

process, frank abscesses can be found with dilated fallopian tubes. Hypo- or hyperechoic tubular structures may be seen adjacent to the uterus. Both MRI and CT easily reveal adnexal disease and pelvic fluid collections.

SELECTED REFERENCES

Ha KH, Lim GY, Cha ES, et al. MR imaging of tubo-ovarian abscess. Acta Radiol. 1995; 36: 510–514.

Langer JE, Dinsmore BJ. Computed tomographic evaluation of benign and inflammatory disorders of the female pelvis. Radiol Clin North Am. 1992; 183: 831–842.

Bulas DI, Ahlstrom PA, Sivit CJ, et al. Pelvic inflammatory disease in the adolescent: comparison of transabdominal and transvaginal sonographic evaluation. Radiology. 1992; 183: 435–439.

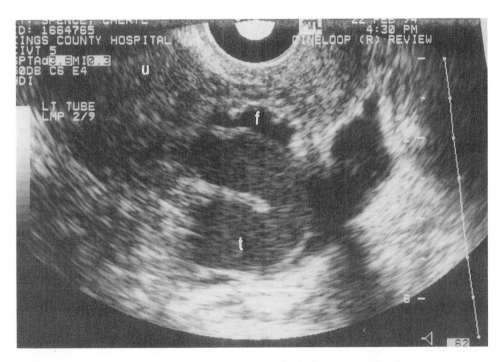

Figure 4–32 Tubo-ovarian abscess. Transvaginal ultrasonography shows a tortuous, dilated, debris-filled fallopian tube (**t**) and free pelvic fluid in the pelvic cul-de-sac (**f**). The normal uterus (**u**) is seen anterior to the abscess.

4.22 HEPATIC ABSCESS

In adults, most pyogenic intrahepatic abscesses occur as an extension of infection through the biliary tree. Hematogenous spread from the portal vein or hepatic artery and contiguous spread from adjacent areas are less common. A gram-negative organism is usually responsible. Symptoms include fever, chills, abdominal pain, nausea, vomiting, jaundice, and pleuritic chest pain. Many patients have abnormal liver function tests. Management consists of parenteral antibiotics combined with percutaneous or surgical drainage.

CT, ultrasound, and MRI are the modalities used for the diagnosis and evaluation of hepatic abscesses. On CT, the lesions are usually of low attenuation and the thickened walls are enhanced after the administration of contrast. Septations and papillary projections may be seen internally. Approximately 80% occur in the right lobe of the liver. Air can be found in approximately 20% of lesions.

MRI offers no additional specificity over CT imaging. T_2-imaging displays high signal, representing the increased water content of the abscess. T_1-weighted images may show internal septations. Ultrasound shows an area of decreased echogenicity, representing the intrahepatic fluid collection. If gas or septations are present, internal echoes are generated.

Amoebic abscesses are rare in the United States. The responsible organism, *Entamoeba histolytica,* is thought to enter the liver through the portal vein, and lesions tend to be located peripherally. CT and ultrasound findings are similar to pyogenic abscesses, although there is a tendency for amoebic abscesses to be unilocular. Echinococcal infection (also known as cysticercosis or hydatid disease) are endemic to sheep-raising populations, and can cause cysts within the liver. Calcifications can be seen in the walls of these low-attenuation lesions on CT. A detached cyst wall can occasionally be seen floating within the cyst ("water lily" sign).

SELECTED REFERENCES

Seeto RK, Rockey DC. Percutaneous management of hepatic abscess: a perspective by interventional radiologists. J Vasc Interv Radiol. 1997; 75: 241–247.

Barreda R, Ros PR. Diagnostic imaging of liver abscess. Crit Rev Diagn Imaging. 1992; 33: 29–58.

Donovan AJ, Yellin AE, Ralls PW. Hepatic abscess. World J Surg. 1991; 23: 162–169.

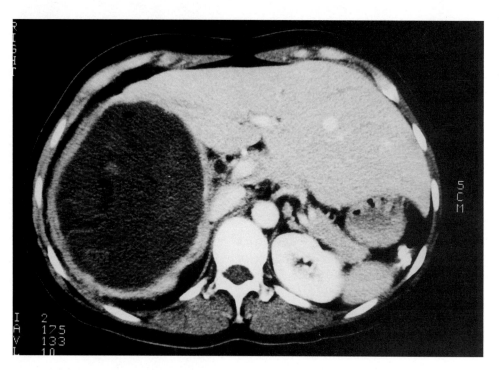

Figure 4–33 Echinococcal hepatic abscess. CT shows a well-demarcated low-density cyst containing internal septations.

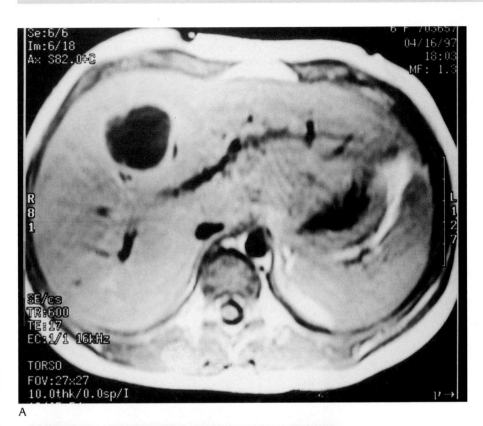

A

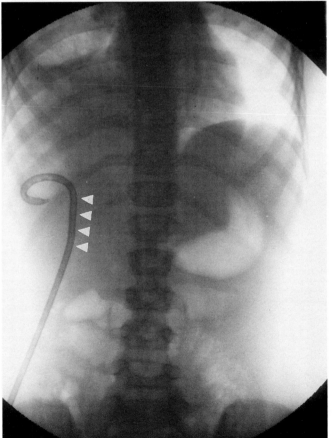

B

Figure 4–34A, B Hepatic abscess. T_1-weighted MRI through the liver reveals a low-signal round mass within the quadrate lobe (**A**). Needle aspiration was consistent with an abscess, which was treated by placement of a percutaneous drainage catheter (**B**, arrowheads).

4.23 HEPATIC LACERATION

Lacerations of the liver parenchyma occur as a result of blunt or penetrating trauma. Grades 1 and 2 injuries, defined as focal tears confined to the parenchyma and not extending to the liver capsule or vascular or biliary structures, can generally be managed conservatively. However, more severe injuries (grades 3 and 4) or those associated with significant intrahepatic or perihepatic bleeding will often need definitive treatment. Both computed tomography and ultrasound can accurately assess the extent of a liver injury. When CT reveals multiple solid organ injuries with associated hemoperitoneum, the location of a higher attenuation "sentinel clot" will often identify the actively bleeding injury. In hemodynamically stable patients with grade 3 or 4 hepatic lacerations and no other injury requiring urgent laparotomy, angiography is the modality of choice to identify a hepatic arterial injury. Selective transcatheter coil embolization of the affected vessel will prevent further bleeding in nearly all cases. Angiographic evaluation of the aorta and of splenic, pelvic, or other abdominal injuries can be simultaneously performed, and additional selective embolization done if necessary.

SELECTED REFERENCES

Davis KA, Brody JM, Cioffi WG. Computed tomography in blunt hepatic trauma. Arch Surg. 1996; 46: 255–260.

Becker CD, Gal I, Baer HU, Vock P. Blunt hepatic trauma in adults: correlation of CT injury grading with outcome. Radiology. 1996; 201: 215–220.

Padhani AR, Watson CJ, Calne RY, Dixon AK. Computed tomography in blunt abdominal trauma: an analysis of clinical management and radiological findings. Clin Radiol. 1992; 46: 304–310.

Hagiwara A, Yukioka T, Ohta S, et al. Nonsurgical management of patients with blunt hepatic injury: efficacy of transcatheter arterial embolization. AJR. 1997; 169: 1151–1156.

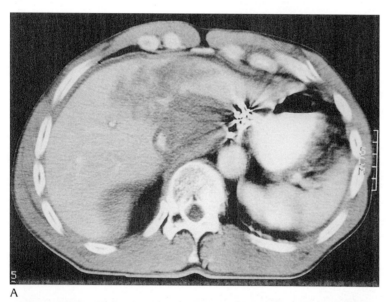

A

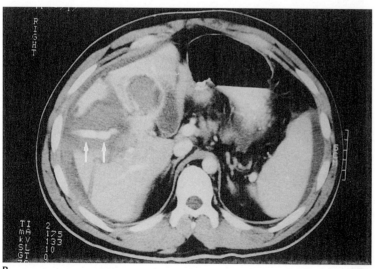

B

Figure 4–35A–D Hepatic laceration. CT images (**A,B**) show low-attenuation fluid within both lobes of the liver, extending to the porta hepatis. There is active extravasation of contrast (**B**, arrows) into the subcapsular space and peritoneum. Angiography confirms the active bleeding (**C**, arrowheads), which was successfully controlled by transcatheter embolization (**D**). Embolization coils are seen in the affected right hepatic arterial branch (open arrow).

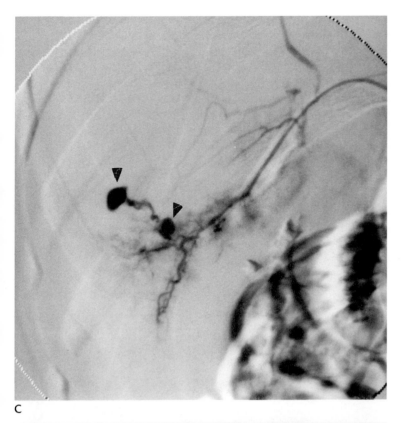

C

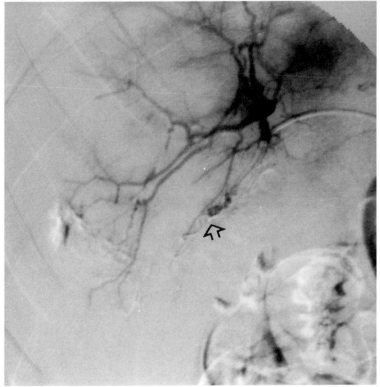

D

4.24 SPLENIC INJURY

Splenic injuries occur in approximately 25% of all patients with major blunt abdominal trauma. The most common clinical findings include evidence of systemic blood loss and left upper quadrant pain. Associated findings are rib fractures, liver injury, pancreatic injury, and pneumothorax.

Initial ultrasound evaluation of the spleen as part of a screening "FAST" (focused abdominal sonography for trauma) examination is becoming increasingly routine in major trauma centers. Lacerations, perisplenic blood, and free intraperitoneal blood can all be recognized with this technique. Contrast-enhanced CT, however, remains the modality of choice for the complete evaluation of splenic injury, and a CT of the abdomen should be performed on all hemodynamically stable patients suspected of having an abdominal injury. CT findings of splenic injury include splenic lacerations, perisplenic hematoma, subcapsular hematoma, splenic infarcts, splenic ruptures, and active hemorrhage. Serial CT scans obtained after blunt abdominal trauma will often show an increase in the volume of the spleen, most likely caused by adrenergic stimulation. This increase, however, is not predictive of clinical deterioration or impending splenic rupture.

Angiographic findings of splenic injury include active extravasation, hypovascular areas representing splenic fractures, lacerations or infarcts, parenchymal compression from subcapsular hematomas, and pseudoaneurysm formation. Therapy using proximal splenic artery embolization is an alternative to splenectomy in patients with ongoing hemorrhage, and can avoid splenectomy in 85–90% of cases.

SELECTED REFERENCES

Sclafani SJ, Shaftan GW, Scalea TM, et al. Nonoperative salvage of computed tomography-diagnosed splenic injuries: utilization of angiography for triage and embolization for hemostasis. J Trauma. 1995; 39: 818–825.

Williams RA, Black JJ, Sinow RM, Wilson SE. Computed tomography-assisted management of splenic trauma. Am J Surg. 1997; 32: 276–279.

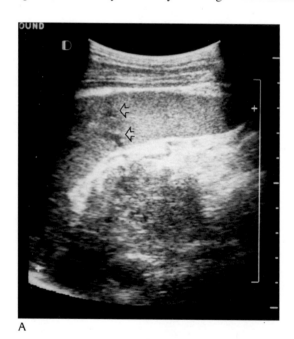

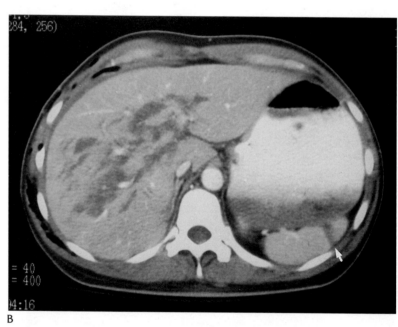

A   B

Figure 4–36A, B Splenic and hepatic injury. Ultrasound (**A**) performed as part of a FAST examination identifies a linear hypoechoic area within the spleen (open arrows). CT on the same patient (**B**) shows both the splenic injury (white arrow) and an associated hepatic laceration.

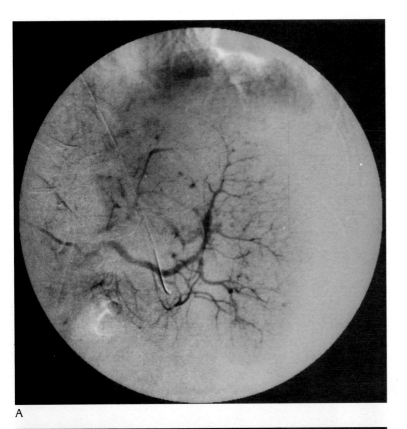

A

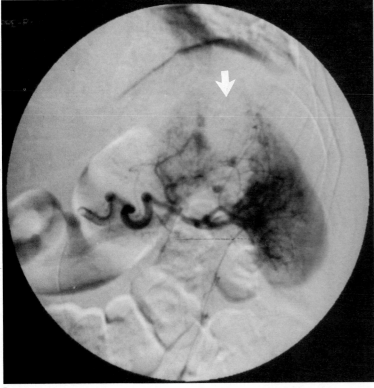

B

Figure 4–37A, B Splenic injury. Selective splenic angiography in two patients with splenic injury reveal multiple areas of punctate bleeding ("starry sky pattern," **A**) and frank extravasation with an associated splenic fracture (**B**, arrow).

4.25 RENAL INJURY

Significant injury following trauma to the kidney is unusual. Most injuries are either grade 1 (contusions) or grade 2 (minor lacerations). Imaging is reserved for patients with significant microscopic or gross hematuria. Intravenous pyelography lacks sufficient sensitivity in most series to be a useful screening examination. Computed tomography and ultrasound scanning can accurately identify parenchymal injuries as well as injuries to other organs. Renal contusions appear as low attenuation or hypoechoic regions within the kidney, whereas lacerations are seen as linear or stellate defects. In grade 2 injuries, the laceration is confined to the renal parenchyma, whereas in grade 3 (major laceration) injuries there is extension to the renal pelvis. Hyperdense perinephric hematoma or areas of nonenhancement on a contrast-enhanced scan may warrant angiography to identify an injury to the vascular pedicle (grade 4 injury). While active extravasation may be treated using transcatheter em-

bolization, major traumatic arterial occlusions often warrant partial or complete nephrectomy. Iatrogenic renal injury, i.e., occurring after renal biopsy, can usually be managed conservatively or with catheter-directed embolization.

SELECTED REFERENCES

Leppaniemi A, Lamminen A, Tervahartiala P, et al. MRI and CT in blunt renal trauma: an update. Semin Ultrasound CT MR. 1997; 18: 129–135.

Miller KS, McAninch JW. Radiographic assessment of renal trauma: our 15-year experience. J Urol. 1995; 146: 352–355.

Mansi MK, Alkhudair WK. Conservative management with percutaneous intervention of major blunt renal injuries. Am J Emerg Med. 1997; 15: 633–637.

Fanney DR, Casillas J, Murphy BJ. CT in the diagnosis of renal trauma. Radiographics. 1990; 46: 29–40.

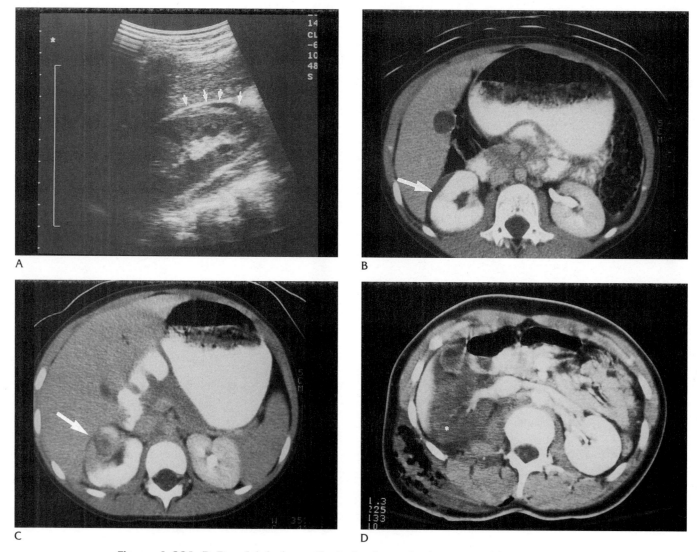

Figure 4–38A–D Renal injuries. Grade 1 subcapsular hematoma (short arrows) on FAST ultrasound (**A**) and subsequent CT (large arrow, **B**), grade 2/3 intraparenchymal hemorrhage (arrow) on CT (**C**), and grade 4 parenchymal infarct (asterisk) due to renal artery avulsion (**D**) as seen on CT.

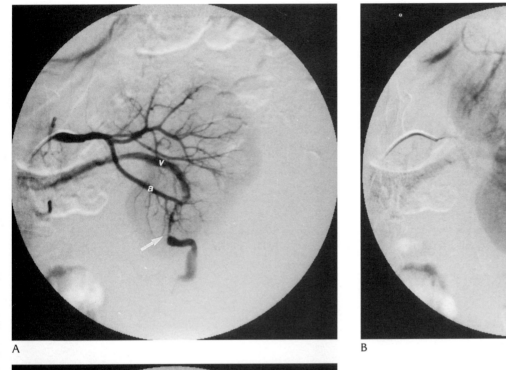

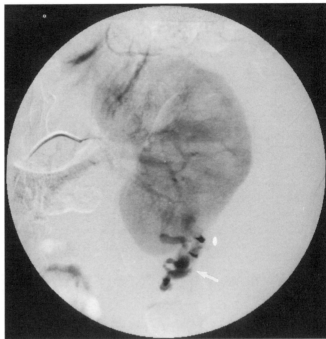

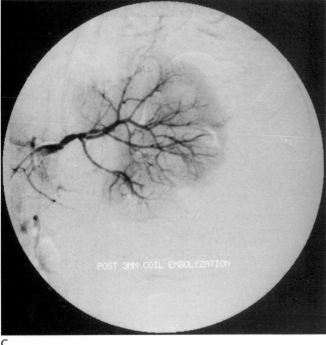

Figure 4–39A–C Renal injury after renal biopsy. Early (**A**) and late (**B**) images from a selective left renal arteriogram reveal an arteriovenous fistula (**a** represents artery; **v,** vein) and active hemorrhage from a lower pole segmental vessel (arrow). After catheter-directed embolization, the fistula is occluded and bleeding is no longer evident (**C**). Perfusion to most of the renal parenchyma is preserved.

4.26 PELVIC FRACTURES AND HEMATOMAS

Pelvic fractures are a potentially life-threatening result of major trauma, and are frequently accompanied by nonorthopedic injuries to the gastrointestinal tract, genitourinary system, central nervous system, and vascular system. Initial management of pelvic fractures should be directed at preventing life-threatening hemorrhage.

Plain radiographs are the initial modality used for evaluating a patient with suspected pelvic fracture. Although routine radiographs are helpful, studies have shown that up to one third of pelvic fractures detected by CT are missed on conventional radiographs. This makes CT an essential element in the diagnosis and preoperative planning of pelvic fractures. In addition, CT can easily evaluate for injury to pelvic organs and pelvic hematomas.

Patients with large pelvic hematomas or who are hemodynamically unstable should undergo emergent arteriography. The superior gluteal artery is the most frequently injured vessel. Bilateral selective internal iliac arteriography is necessary to exclude arterial hemorrhage. Should an injury be found, the bleeding vessel may be selectively occluded using catheter-directed embolotherapy.

SELECTED REFERENCES

Berg EE, Chebuhar C, Bell RM. Pelvic trauma imaging: a blinded comparison of computed tomography and roentgenograms. J Trauma. 1996; 41: 994–998.

Cerva DS, Mirvis SE, Shanmuganathan K, et al. Detection of bleeding in patients with major pelvic fractures: value of contrast-enhanced CT. AJR. 1996; 166: 131–135.

Agolini SF, Shah K, Jaffe J, et al. Arterial embolization is a rapid and effective technique for controlling pelvic fracture hemorrhage. J Trauma. 1997; 43: 395–399.

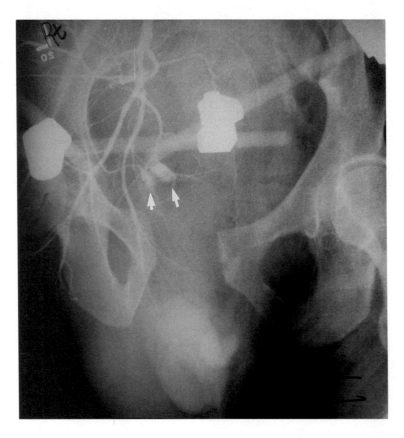

Figure 4–40 Pelvic fracture with hypogastric bleeding. Selective right hypogastric arteriography shows diastasis pubis, an external fixator, and active contrast extravasation from the internal pudendal artery (short arrows).

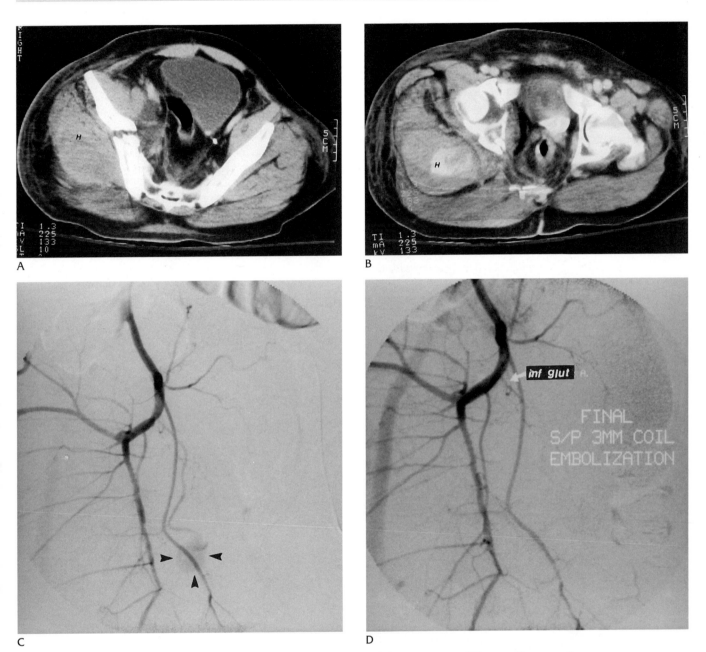

Figure 4–41A–D Pelvic fracture and gluteal hematoma. CT scans from another patient (**A, B**) show multiple fractures of the right iliac wing and acetabulum. A large inferior gluteal hematoma is present (**H**), and appears as high attenuation within the muscle body. On hypogastric arteriography (**C**), there is a pseudoaneurysm of the distal inferior gluteal artery (arrowheads). This was successfully treated with transcatheter coil embolization (**D**).

4.27 BLADDER RUPTURE

Nearly 80% of urinary bladder ruptures are extraperitoneal and occur in association with pelvic fractures. Imaging is reserved for patients with significant hematuria (>50 RBC per high power field), and retrograde cystography is the usual initial diagostic examination. On early filling, the bladder assumes a "pear-shaped" configuration due to compression by surrounding urinoma or pelvic hematoma. Later images and postvoiding films show extravasation of contrast into adjacent fat planes. Intraperitoneal rupture of the dome of the bladder is less common and may be iatrogenic, or the result of minor trauma in a distended bladder. More rarely, spontaneous rupture occurs in association with alcohol or other drug intoxication. On cystography, contrast extravasation is seen to surround bowel loops and fill the paracolic gutters. Both intraperitoneal and extraperitoneal ruptures may be detected when CT scans are performed for evaluation of other injuries. The bladder will usu-

ally appear small, and contrast will be noted outside the bladder. Delayed scans are helpful in identifying the location of the bladder injury. Extraperitoneal rupture can often be managed by prolonged catheter decompression of the bladder.

SELECTED REFERENCES

Rehm CG, Mure AJ, O'Malley KF, Ross SE. Evaluation and treatment of bladder rupture. Semin Urol. 1995; 20: 62–65.

Horstman WG, McClennan BL, Heiken JP. Comparison of computed tomography and conventional cystography for detection of traumatic bladder rupture. Urol Radiol. 1991; 29: 188–193.

Sivit CJ, Cutting JP, Eichelberger MR. CT diagnosis and localization of rupture of the bladder in children with blunt abdominal trauma: significance of contrast material extravasation in the pelvis. AJR. 1995; 20: 1243–1246.

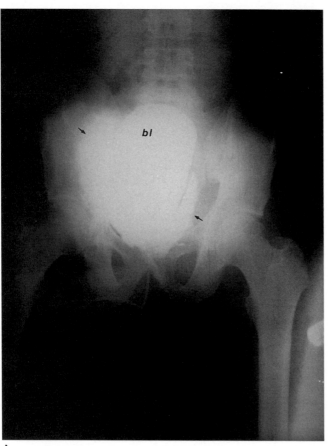

A

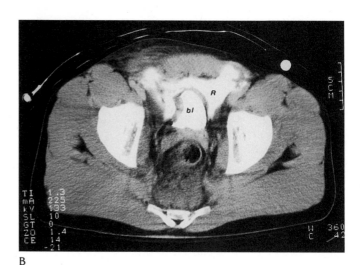

B

Figure 4–42A, B Extraperitoneal bladder rupture. Cystography (**A**) shows contrast (arrows) collecting outside the filled bladder (**bl**). There is resulting bladder compression causing the characteristic "pear-shaped" appearance. A corresponding pelvic CT scan (**B**) displays contrast anterior and lateral to the bladder within the space of Retzius (**R**).

4.28 FREE PERITONEAL FLUID

The accumulation of fluid in the peritoneal cavity is called ascites. The fluid may be a transudate or an exudate. Transudative ascites may result from cirrhosis, congestive heart failure, hypoproteinemia, or venous obstruction. Exudative ascites is associated with trauma, pancreatitis, bowel perforation, and peritonitis. Chylous ascites is due to obstruction or trauma to the thoracic duct. Likewise, urine ascites can occur after trauma or obstruction to the urinary tracts.

The abdominal and the pelvic cavities form a continuum with fluid freely flowing between the two spaces. Small amounts of fluid tend to accumulate in the most dependent locations including the pelvic cul-de-sac and Morison's pouch (the space between the liver and the right kidney). Although large amounts of ascites can be seen on abdominal radiographs, ultrasound and CT are the modality of choice when looking for free peritoneal fluid.

Paracentesis is necessary for determining the precise nature of the ascites. Some clues to the type of fluid can be obtained with CT by evaluating the attenuation of the fluid. Acute blood has an attenuation of approximately 45H (Hounsfield units), whereas serous ascites has an attenuation of approximately −10 to +10H. Fluid is seen on CT as varying density surrounding bowel loops and collecting in dependent spaces.

Ultrasound is excellent for localizing ascites. The sonographic appearance of fluid is variable, depending on its composition. Simple ascites is sonolucent, whereas hemorrhage contains echoes and may contain septations and floating debris.

SELECTED REFERENCES

DeMeo JH, Fulcher AS, Austin RF Jr. Anatomic CT demonstration of the peritoneal spaces, ligaments, and mesenteries: normal and pathologic processes. Radiographics. 1995; 15: 755–770.

Demas BE. Imaging of peritoneal pathology. Curr Opin Radiol. 1992; 4: 124–127.

Thoeni RF. The role of imaging in patients with ascites. AJR. 1995; 165: 16–18.

Ruess L, Frazier AA, Sivit CJ. CT of the mesentery, omentum, and peritoneum in children. Radiographics. 1995; 15: 89–104.

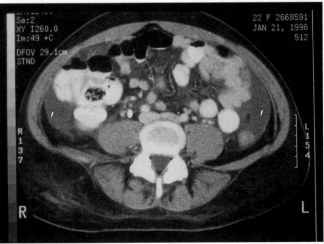

A

B

Figure 4–43A, B Free intraperitoneal fluid. Low-attenuation fluid is noted in Morison's pouch (**M**), surrounding the spleen, and in both paracolic gutters (**f**). Inflammatory changes are incidentally seen within the pancreas.

4.29 PNEUMOPERITONEUM

Pneumoperitoneum represents the extraluminal collection of air within the abdominal cavity. In adults, intraperitoneal gas collections may be benign (after laparoscopy or laparotomy, peritoneal dialysis or lavage), iatrogenic (due to bladder or intestinal rupture during endoscopy), or secondary to an underlying pathologic process (eg, abscess, hollow viscus rupture, extension of a pneumothorax). Postoperative pneumoperitoneum resolves rapidly; nearly all intraperitoneal air is resorbed by 1 week.

Plain film findings of pneumoperitoneum include air outlining both sides of the bowel (Rigler's sign), gas outlining the falciform ligament in the medial right upper quadrant of the abdomen, gas outlining the peritoneal cavity (football sign), triangular air pockets between bowel loops, or gas localized to the right upper quadrant. Upright PA and lateral chest radiographs may improve the detection of small intraperitoneal gas collections by revealing air accumulation under the diaphragm. When this is not possible, a left lateral decubitus abdominal film will show an air collection lateral to the liver surface, and is more sensitive than supine images. Computed tomography is highly sensitive in detecting small amounts of intraperitoneal air. This sensitivity, however, may result in an occasional false suspicion of bowel rupture, and close clinical observation as well as further contrast studies is advisable to identify an intestinal injury before surgical exploration.

SELECTED REFERENCES

Woodring JH, Heiser MJ. Detection of pneumoperitoneum on chest radiographs: comparison of upright lateral and posteroanterior projections. AJR. 1995; 11: 45–47.

Levine MS, Scheiner JD, Rubesin SE, et al. Diagnosis of pneumoperitoneum on supine abdominal radiographs. AJR. 1991; 156: 731–735.

Kane NM, Francis IR, Burney RE, et al. Traumatic pneumoperitoneum. Implications of computed tomography diagnosis. Invest Radiol. 1991; 26: 574–578.

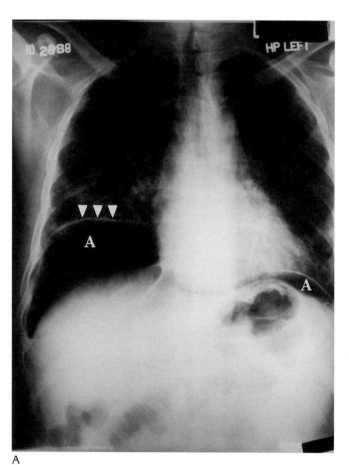

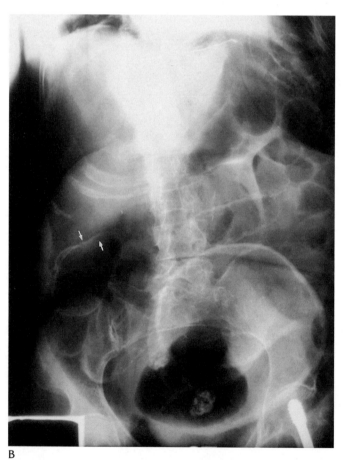

A

B

Figure 4–44A, B Pneumoperitoneum. Plain film of the abdomen (**A**) shows free air under the diaphragm (**A** represents air; arrowheads, diaphragm). Air outlining both walls of the bowel, Rigler's sign, is noted in another patient (**B**, arrows).

4.30 HYDRONEPHROSIS/URINARY TRACT OBSTRUCTION

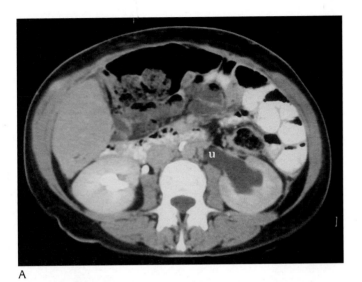

A

Dilatation of the renal collecting system is termed hydronephrosis, and is representative of urinary tract obstruction. Common causes of obstruction include impacted renal stones, pelvic malignancy, recent pelvic surgery, bladder outlet obstruction (prostate cancer or benign prostatic hyperplasia), and renal sepsis. Ultrasound and CT are the modalities of choice when evaluating for hydronephrosis.

Hydronephrosis produces separation of normal sinus echogenicity by anechoic urine within the renal calyces. These dilated anechoic calyces are seen to connect to the renal pelvis, which is also dilated. Visualization of this connection helps distinguish hydronephrosis from parapelvic cysts. CT readily shows the dilated collecting system, either with or without contrast. Dependent layering of unopacified urine over the heavier contrast material is commonly observed. The affected kidney may show delayed contrast excretion as compared with the opposite side. CT scanning is also effective in determining both the level and cause of obstruction by demonstrating calculi, tumor, or an extrinsic mass.

SELECTED REFERENCES

Koelliker SL, Cronan JJ. Acute urinary tract obstruction. Imaging update. Urol Clin North Am. 1997; 24: 571–582.

Chen MY, Zagoria RJ, Dyer RB. Radiologic findings in acute urinary tract obstruction. J Emerg Med. 1997; 15: 339–343.

Haddad MC, Sharif HS, Shahed MS, et al. Renal colic: diagnosis and outcome. Radiology. 1992; 184: 83–88.

O'Malley ME, Soto JA, Yucel EK, Hussain S. MR urography: evaluation of a three-dimensional fast spin-echo technique in patients with hydronephrosis. AJR. 1997; 168: 387–392.

B

Figure 4–45A, B Hydronephrosis. CT scan (**A**) and ultrasound (**B**) reveal dilatation of the renal-collecting system (**c** represents calyces) and associated proximal hydroureter (**u**).

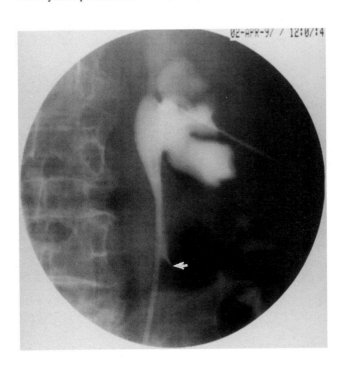

Figure 4–46 Hydronephrosis. Blunting of the calyces is observed on an antegrade pyelogram. There is urinary obstruction due to a transitional cell tumor of the ureter, resulting in a meniscus and "goblet sign" at the point of ureteral occlusion (arrow). An internal ureteral stent has been inserted across the obstruction.

4.31 SMALL BOWEL OBSTRUCTION

Mechanical small bowel obstruction (SBO) occurs most frequently in adults because of intra-abdominal adhesions that develop after previous surgery or peritonitis. Other causes include hernias, volvulus, intussusception, and tumor. In children, malrotation, Meckel's diverticulum and appendicitis are further potential causes of SBO. Flat plate, upright, and decubitus radiographs of the abdomen (KUB series) frequently are diagnostic. Plain film findings are dilated small bowel loops with multiple air-fluid levels (at least 3 air-fluid levels of at least 5 cm in length), and stretched mucosal folds. Little or no gas may be seen in the colon in cases of complete obstruction. Air projecting over the groin may be indicative of an inguinal hernia, and a calcification in the lower right abdomen suggests the diagnosis of gallstone ileus (in adults) or appendicitis (in children). Upper GI series using barium will frequently reveal the level of obstruction as an abrupt cutoff in the contrast column. With partial obstructions, a marked change in the intestinal caliber will be evident distal to the point of obstruction. Air or contrast filling of the biliary tree may be found in cases of gallstone ileus. Spiral computed tomography has emerged as an important diagnostic tool in the evaluation of patients with suspected SBO, and can detect cases of bowel strangulation, ischemia, or perforation. Findings include wall thickening, dilatation, changes in luminal diameter, a laminated pattern of enhancement of the bowel wall ("target sign"), and absence of contrast opacification distal to the obstruction. Recently, MRI using rapid sequence protocols has also shown promise for diagnosing the etiology of bowel obstruction.

Recent studies indicate that formation of abdominal adhesions is inhibited by antibodies to transforming growth factor β1. These results indicate that specifically reducing levels of TFG-β1 alone can be effective in preventing abdominal adhesions and thus prevent bowel obstruction.

SELECTED REFERENCES

Maglinte DD, Reyes BL, Harmon BH, et al. Reliability and role of plain film radiography and CT in the diagnosis of small-bowel obstruction. AJR. 1996; 167: 1451–1455.

Regan F, Beall DP, Bohman ME, et al. Fast MR imaging and the detection of small-bowel obstruction. AJR. 1998; 170: 1465–1469.

Jabra AA, Fishman EK. Small bowel obstruction in the pediatric patient: CT evaluation. Abdom Imaging. 1997; 22: 466–470.

Balthazar EJ, Birnbaum BA, Megibow AJ, et al. Closed-loop and strangulating intestinal obstruction: CT signs. Radiology. 1992; 185: 769–775.

Lucas PA, Warejcka DJ, Young HE, Lee BY. Formation of abdominal adhesions is inhibited by antibodies to transforming growth factor beta. J Surg Res. 1996; 65: 135–138.

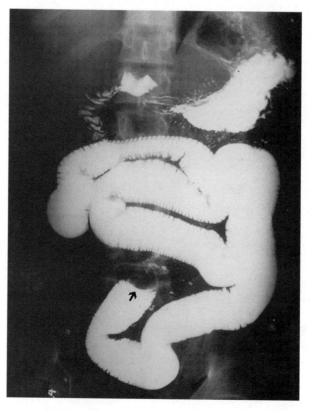

Figure 4–47 Small bowel obstruction. On a supine film, multiple air-filled, dilated loops of small bowel are seen. No colonic gas is present.

Figure 4–48 Small bowel obstruction. An upper GI series and small bowel follow-through show jejunal dilatation. An obstructing mass is present in the distal jejunum (arrow).

4.32 LARGE BOWEL OBSTRUCTION

Hospital admissions for colonic obstruction are not uncommon. Symptoms of large bowel obstruction (LBO) tend to develop slowly and include abdominal distention, abdominal pain, and constipation or watery diarrhea. Causes of mechanical LBO include malignancy, diverticulitis, inflammatory bowel disease, fecal impaction, volvulus, and hernias. Unlike small bowel obstructions, adhesions are rarely found to be the cause of colonic obstruction. Colonic obstructions also produce less fluid and electrolyte disturbances than SBO.

The radiographic appearance of LBO depends on the competency of the ileocecal valve. When the ileocecal valve is competent, the colon becomes markedly dilated with air, and there is little air in the small intestine. With an incompetent valve, both the colon and small bowel become distended. Depending on the location of the obstruction, an abrupt "cutoff" of the air column may be seen.

When plain films suggest colonic obstruction, the diagnosis should be confirmed by endoscopy or barium enema. Oral barium should never be given because it may solidify proximal to the obstruction and cause further complication. Prompt decompression is mandatory to prevent perforation, which becomes more likely as the colonic diameter approaches 10 cm. On a barium enema, different disease processes can have similar appearances. However, the examination will occasionally allow a definitive diagnosis of the cause of obstruction. Malignancies classically produce "apple core" lesions, whereas strictures, fistulas, and diverticuli are classically seen with diverticulitis.

SELECTED REFERENCES

Frager D, Rovno HD, Baer JW, et al. Prospective evaluation of colonic obstruction with computed tomography. Abdom Imaging. 1998; 23: 141–146.

Chapman AH, McNamara M, Porter G. The acute contrast enema in suspected large bowel obstruction: value and technique. Clin Radiol. 1992; 46: 273–278.

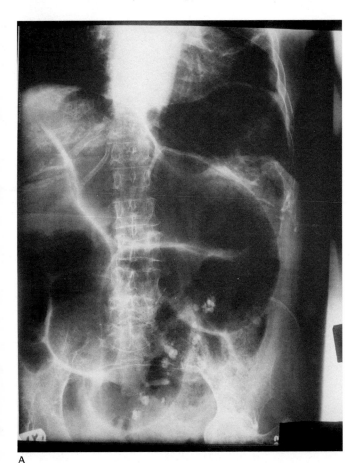

A

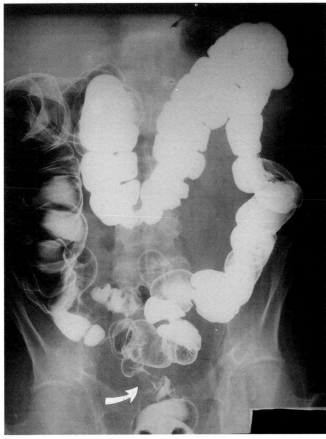

B

Figure 4–49A, B Large bowel obstruction. Dilated colon (**A**) is noted on an abdominal radiograph (KUB). A barium enema of a different patient (**B**) shows an obstructing "apple-core" mass in the rectosigmoid colon (curved arrow).

4.33 COLONIC VOLVULUS

Volvulus of the large bowel may involve either the cecum or sigmoid colon. Cecal volvulus occurs in association with intestinal malrotation or may be caused by an abnormally long cecal mesentery (cecal bascule). Abdominal radiographs show distention of the cecum in a reniform pattern extending to the left upper quadrant of the abdomen; dilatation exceeding 15 cm in diameter requires urgent surgical or image-guided decompression to avoid the high risk for cecal perforation. Sigmoid volvulus generally occurs in elderly, bedridden, demented patients, or in those receiving constipating medications. Torsion occurs along the mesenteric axis of the sigmoid colon, producing a markedly dilated sigmoid loop extending from the left side of the pelvis toward the diaphragm and containing air-fluid levels. On supine radiographs, the apposition of the mesenteric surfaces of the distended sigmoid results in a characteristic "coffee bean sign." In both sigmoid and cecal volvulus, barium studies will reveal a beak-like appearance of the contrast at the point of obstruction. Computed tomography is useful in diagnosing equivocal cases of sigmoid volvulus, because the dilated sigmoid will have a unique whorl-like pattern around the mesocolon and mesenteric vasculature.

SELECTED REFERENCES

Catalano O. Computed tomographic appearance of sigmoid volvulus. Abdom Imaging. 1996; 21: 314–317.

Theuer C, Cheadle WG. Volvulus of the colon. Am Surg. 1991; 57: 145–150.

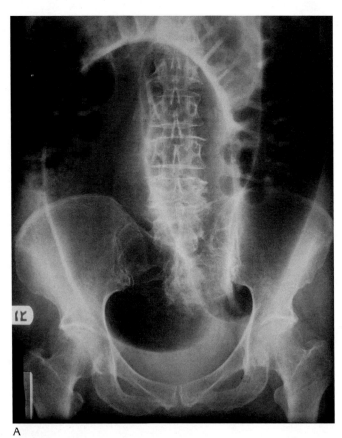

A

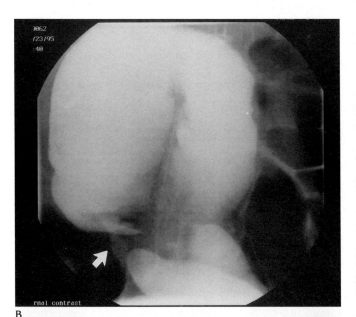

B

C

Figure 4–50A–C Sigmoid volvulus. A KUB radiograph (**A**) shows a dilated sigmoid colon directed toward the right upper quadrant, which looks like a "coffee-bean" configuration. A beak is noted at the point of torsion (arrows) on a gastrografin enema (**B, C**).

4.34 INTUSSUSCEPTION

Intussusception represents an invagination of a loop of bowel into adjacent bowel. The invaginated bowel is called the intussusceptum; the surrounding bowel is called the intussuscepiens. Three quarters of intussusceptions occur in infants younger than 2 years of age. In children, 90% of intussusceptions have no pathologic cause. Intussusceptions resulting from pathologic conditions usually occur after age 4. Pathologic origins that may result in intussusception include Meckel's diverticulum, polyps, cancer, and appendiceal inflammation. Patients with sprue and cystic fibrosis also have a predisposition to developing intussusception. Greater than 90% of intussusceptions in children are ileocolic or ileoileocolic. Symptoms include abdominal pain, fever, vomiting, and "currant jelly" stools. This condition should be considered a pediatric emergency and a surgeon contacted immediately.

If there is no clinical evidence of peritonitis and there is no free air in the abdomen on radiographs, a barium enema may be performed both for diagnostic purposes and with the intent of decompressing the intussusception. On the barium enema, the intussusception typically appears as a "coil-spring" with barium between the inner and outer loops of bowel. Therapeutic reduction of the intussusception occurs in 65–75% of cases. Pneumatic reduction (using gas instead of barium) is also possible, which has reported success rates as high as 80–90%.

CT and ultrasound can also be used to diagnose intussusception. CT will demonstrate an inner loop with its mesentery surrounded by the outer loop. A unique "doughnut" appearance is apparent on axial sonographic images. In adults, CT is the imaging method of choice because it reveals an underlying malignant lesion in approximately one half of cases. In these cases, surgical resection of the intussusception without decompression is preferable.

SELECTED REFERENCES

Azar T, Berger DL. Adult intussusception. Ann Surg. 1997; 226: 134–138.

Gayer G, Apster S, Hofmann C, et al. Intussusception in adults: CT diagnosis. Clin Radiol. 1998; 53: 53–57.

Ratcliffe JF, Fong S, Cheong I, O'Connell P. The plain abdominal film in intussusception: the accuracy and incidence of radiograph signs. Pediatr Radiol. 1992; 22: 110–111.

Del-Pozo G, Albillos JC, Tejedor D. Intussusception: US findings with pathologic correlation—the crescent-in-doughnut sign. Radiology. 1996; 199: 688–692.

Shiels WE II, Maves CK, Hedlund GL, Kirks DR. Air enema for diagnosis and reduction of intussusception: clinical experience and pressure correlates. Radiology. 1991; 181: 169–172.

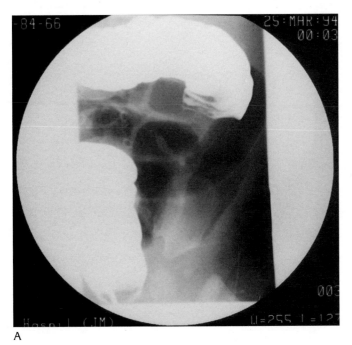

A

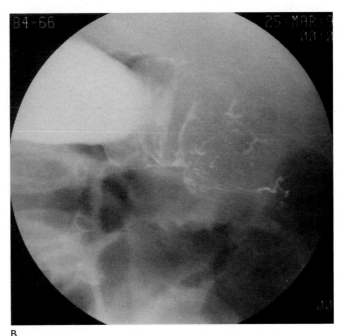

B

Figure 4–51A, B Intussusseption. Early (**A**) and late (**B**) images from a barium enema (the patient is prone so that the ascending colon is on the right). There is obstruction of the ascending colon with a "coil-spring" appearance due to contrast layering around the intussusceptum.

4.35 OVARIAN TORSION

Ovarian torsion is caused by rotation around the vascular pedicle, depriving the ovary of arterial blood and preventing venous drainage. This causes ovarian congestion, and can lead to hemorrhage and infarction. Torsion usually occurs during childhood or the teenage years. Although torsion may occur in normal ovaries, it is more commonly associated with ovarian tumors and cysts. Patients present with pelvic pain, nausea, and vomiting. Occasionally, a palpable adnexal mass is present. Ovarian torsion is a surgical emergency and requires prompt intervention.

Duplex ultrasound is an excellent way of evaluating patients with suspected ovarian torsion. On ultrasound, a unilaterally enlarged ovary, which contains multiple cortical follicles, is considered specific for ovarian torsion. The follicles are seen as round hypoechoic collections at the periphery of the gland. Color flow and duplex Doppler sonography reveal absent blood flow within the ovary, confirming the diagnosis.

SELECTED REFERENCES

Meyer JS, Harmon CM, Harty MP, et al. Ovarian torsion: clinical and imaging presentation in children. J Pediatr Surg. 1995; 30: 1433–1436.

Jain KA. Magnetic resonance imaging finding in ovarian torsion. Magn Reson Imaging. 1995; 13: 111–113.

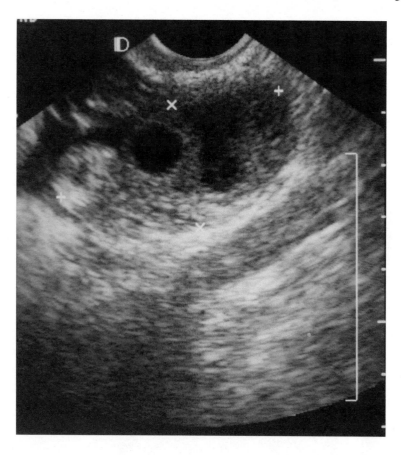

Figure 4–52 Ovarian torsion. Enlargement, heterogeneity, and cystic changes are observed in the right ovary on transvaginal sonography. No flow was seen on Doppler ultrasonography.

4.36 TESTICULAR TORSION

Testicular torsion is a surgical emergency and the most common cause of an acutely painful, swollen scrotum. Other differential possibilities are epididymitis, epididymo-orchitis, acute hydrocele, testicular abscess, and strangulated hernia. Torsion is more common in children, but accounts for up to 20% of scrotal disease in postpubertal men. A history of prior orchiopexy for undescended testes increases the risk of torsion 10-fold. If surgery is performed within 6 hours after the onset of pain, the testicular salvage rate is between 80% and 100%. This rate decreases to 20% as the time from onset of symptoms to surgery increases beyond 12 hours.

The differentiation between testicular torsion and epididymo-orchitis can be difficult on the basis of clinical examination and laboratory findings. Doppler ultrasonography and radionuclide imaging can help distinguish these two entities. Sonographically, in cases of torsion, the testicle appears enlarged, hypoechoic, and inhomogeneous compared with the unaffected side. An enlarged epididymis and a reactive hydrocele are associated nonspecific findings. Color Doppler imaging of testicular torsion reveals decreased or absent flow in the involved testicle. In contrast, normal or increased flow in the involved testicle is seen in patients with epididymo-orchitis.

The scintigraphic findings of testicular torsion depend on the time that has elapsed since the patient presented with severe pain. In early torsion, flow images may not show any significant asymmetry. On the tissue phase image, decreased activity may be seen in the region of the involved testicle. It is important to bear in mind that a normal result from a testicular scintigram in early testicular torsion does not rule out its presence, because compensatory changes may obscure the decreased uptake. Later in the course of torsion, an area of decreased activity representing the ischemic testicle is seen, which is surrounded by a rim of increased activity representing hyperemia. If testicular torsion cannot be definitively ruled out by Doppler ultrasonography or radionuclide imaging, immediate surgical exploration of the scrotum should be performed.

SELECTED REFERENCES

Melloul M, Paz A, Lask D, et al. The value of radionuclide scrotal imaging in the diagnosis of acute testicular torsion. Br J Urol. 1995; 76: 628–631.

Burks DD, Markey BJ, Burkhard TK, et al. Suspected testicular torsion and ischemia: evaluation with color Doppler sonography. Radiology. 1990; 175: 815–821.

Suzer O, Ozcan H, Kupeli S, Gheiler EL. Color Doppler imaging in the diagnosis of the acute scrotum. Eur Urol. 1997; 199: 457–461.

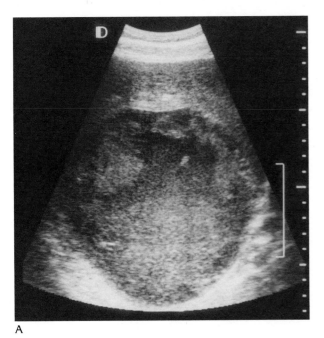

A

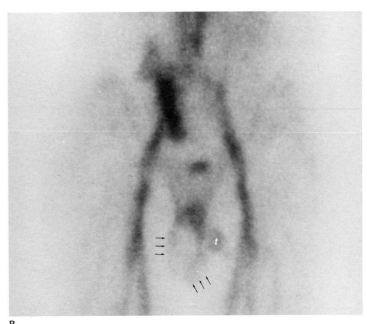

B

Figure 4–53A, B Testicular torsion. A testicular ultrasound (**A**) shows edema and inhomogeneity of the right testicle. A small amount of fluid (hydrocele) is present. A radionuclide testicular scan (**B**) reveals a cold defect in the region of the right hemiscrotum with surrounding hyperemia (rim sign, arrows). The left testicle appears normal (**t**).

4.37 ECTOPIC PREGNANCY

Ectopic pregnancies account for approximately 1.4% of gestations, and are responsible for up to 15% of maternal deaths. Risk factors include any tubal abnormality that can prevent passage of the zygote, including pelvic inflammatory disease, previous tubal pregnancy, intrauterine devices, prior tubal reconstructive surgery, and increased maternal age. Approximately 95% of ectopic pregnancies occur within the ampullary or isthmic portions of the uterus. The classic clinical triad of pain, abnormal vaginal bleeding, and a palpable adnexal mass is present in only 45% of patients with ectopic pregnancy. Other symptoms and signs include amenorrhea and cervical "motion" pain. A serum test for the β subunit of HCG should be performed on all patients in whom ectopic pregnancy is considered. A positive pregnancy test in a patient with appropriate symptoms mandates that the patient have a pelvic ultrasound to identify the location of the gestational sac. Patients with ectopic pregnancy will have a complex, cystic, echogenic adnexal mass. While there may be hormonally induced thickening of the endometrium (a pseudogestational sac), the double decidual sign seen in normal intrauterine pregnancy will not be present.

Endovaginal sonograms can reveal an intrauterine pregnancy earlier than a transabdominal study. The demonstration of a live embryo in the adnexa is diagnostic of ectopic pregnancy. Nonspecific sonographic findings include free pelvic fluid and an empty uterine cavity in the presence of an elevated titer for the β subunit of HCG. The presence of an intrauterine pregnancy essentially rules out the possibility of an ectopic pregnancy (concurrent intrauterine and ectopic pregnancies occur at a rate of 1 in 7000).

SELECTED REFERENCES

Penzia AS, Huang PL. Imaging in ectopic pregnancy. J Reprod Med. 1992; 37: 47–53.

Brennan DF. Ectopic pregnancy—Part II: diagnostic procedures and imaging. Acad Emerg Med. 1995; 2: 1090–1097.

Frates MC, Laing FC. Sonographic evaluation of ectopic pregnancy: an update. AJR. 1995; 165: 251–259.

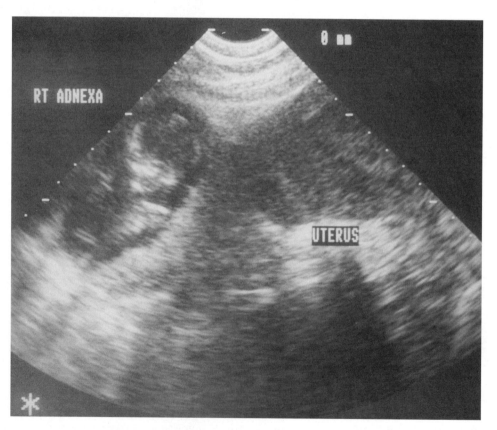

Figure 4–54 Ectopic pregnancy. A fetus is apparent within the right adnexa on a transabdominal ultrasound.

4.38 FOCUSED ABDOMINAL SONOGRAPHY FOR TRAUMA

Patients sustaining severe multiorgan trauma require a prompt diagnosis of all surgically relevant injuries, and are frequently too unstable to tolerate the time or transfer necessary for definitive CT or other radiologic imaging. Focused abdominal sonography for trauma (FAST) studies can be performed in less than 5 minutes in the emergency room or operating room, and have a reported sensitivity and specificity of 88% and 99% for the detection of significant intra-abdominal injury. FAST studies rely on the demonstration of hemoperitoneum, and there is the potential for missing important abdominal injury without associated free fluid. Computed tomography or diagnostic peritoneal lavage should be performed whenever possible on patients with indeterminate sonographic studies or clinical evidence of abdominal injury.

SELECTED REFERENCES

McKenney MG, Martin L, Lentz K, et al. 1000 consecutive ultrasounds for blunt abdominal trauma. J Trauma. 1996; 40: 607–610.

Chiu WC, Cushing BM, Rodriguez A, et al. Abdominal injuries without hemoperitoneum: a potential limitation of focused abdominal sonography for trauma (FAST). J Trauma. 1997; 42: 617–623.

Boulanger BR, Brenneman FD, Kirkpatrick AW, et al. The indeterminate abdominal sonogram in multisystem blunt trauma. J Trauma. 1998; 45: 52–56.

CHAPTER 5

EXTREMITY IMAGING

John H. Rundback, MD

Maurice R. Poplausky, MD

Bok Y. Lee, MD, FACS

5.1 NORMALS

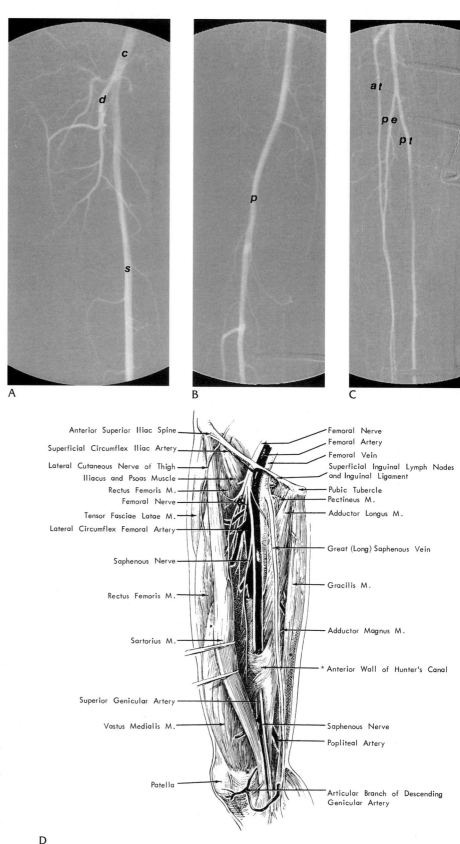

Figure 5–1A–D Normal lower extremity arteriogram at the level of the femoral bifurcation (**A**), popliteal (**B**), and tibial runoff vessels (**C**). **c** represents common femoral artery; **s**, superficial femoral artery; **d**, profunda femoral artery; **p**, popliteal artery; **at**, anterior tibial artery; **pt**, posterior tibial artery; and **pe**, peroneal artery. A corresponding line drawing of the upper thigh (**D**) shows normal vascular anatomy above the knee.

Anterior Superior Iliac Spine

Superficial Circumflex Iliac Artery

Lateral Cutaneous Nerve of Thigh

Iliacus and Psoas Muscle

Rectus Femoris M.

Femoral Nerve

Tensor Fasciae Latae M.

Lateral Circumflex Femoral Artery

Saphenous Nerve

Rectus Femoris M.

Sartorius M.

Superior Genicular Artery

Vastus Medialis M.

Patella

Femoral Nerve

Femoral Artery

Femoral Vein

Superficial Inguinal Lymph Nodes and Inguinal Ligament

Pubic Tubercle

Pectineus M.

Adductor Longus M.

Great (Long) Saphenous Vein

Gracilis M.

Adductor Magnus M.

* Anterior Wall of Hunter's Canal

Saphenous Nerve

Popliteal Artery

Articular Branch of Descending Genicular Artery

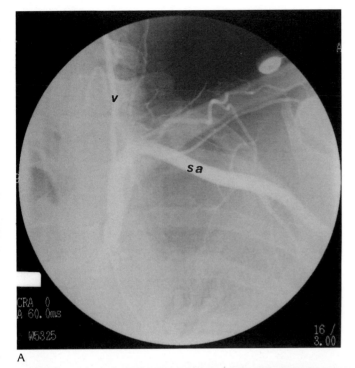

A

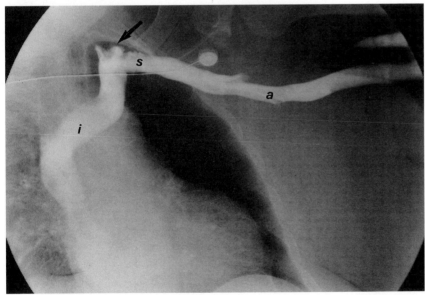

B

Figure 5–2A, B Normal subclavian arteriogram (**A**) and venogram (**B**). **a** represents axillary vein; **s**, subclavian vein; **i**, innominate vein; **sa**, subclavian artery; **v**, vertebral artery. An arrow marks the inflow of the internal jugular vein.

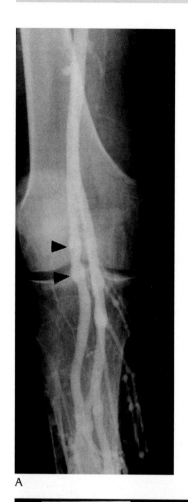

A

Figure 5–3A–C Normal lower extremity venogram (**A**) and venous Doppler (**B, C**). A duplicated popliteal vein and lower superficial femoral vein are noted to be widely patent. Valve cusps are evident as focal areas of venous enlargement (arrowheads). A duplex sonogram shows normal compressibility of the common femoral vein (**v** represents vein; **a**, artery). Flow augmentation during calf-compression is demonstrated using spectral Doppler (**C**).

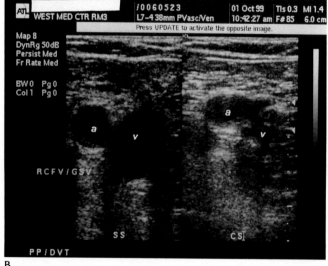

B

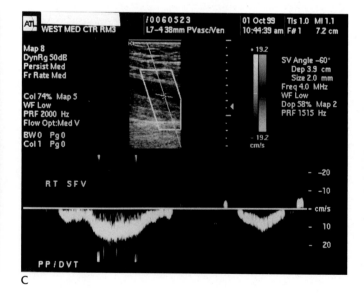

C

5.2 DEEP VENOUS THROMBOSIS

Patients with acute deep venous thrombosis (DVT) of the lower extremities can be asymptomatic, or may present with pain, leg swelling, and rubor. Most thrombi develop in either the valvular sinuses of the calf veins or within the conduit veins. These thrombi can then propagate centrally, and involve the popliteal vein in approximately 20% of cases. The major morbidity associated with lower extremity DVT is pulmonary embolization (PE). Approximately one half of patients with acute DVT have been shown to have pulmonary embolism at the time of initial diagnosis. Treatment options include anticoagulation treatment with low molecular weight or unfractionated heparin, or inferior vena cava (IVC) filter placement in those patients who cannot tolerate anticoagulation or who have recurrent PE despite anticoagulation therapy. More recently, catheter-directed infusion of thrombolytic agents such as urokinase or t-PA have been used in cases of acute proximal (iliofemoral) DVT to dissolve clot, decrease the extent of valvular damage, and reduce the incidence of chronic venous insufficiency causing postphlebitic syndrome.

Duplex imaging has become the initial test of choice for diagnosing DVT, and has an accuracy of approximately 95%. Diagnostic criteria include the visualization of echogenic thrombus in the vein, loss of compressibility, venous distention, loss of flow augmentation, and absence of the normal respiratory variability on Doppler imaging. Contrast venography remains the reference standard for confirming or excluding the presence

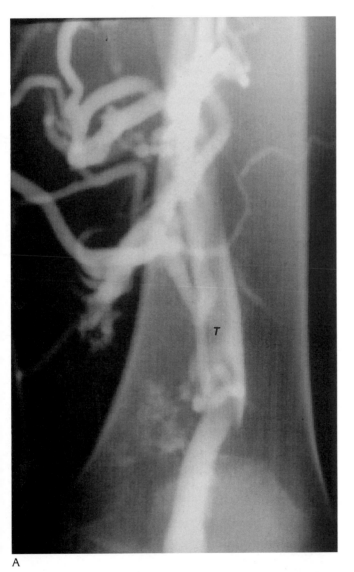

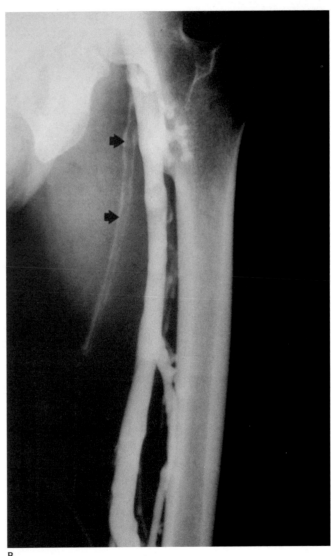

A

B

Figure 5–4A, B Acute deep venous thrombosis (DVT). A lower extremity venogram (**A**) shows an acute thrombus (**T**) within the popliteal vein. A venogram in another patient (**B**) reveals a linear filling defect within the greater saphenous vein of the left leg (short arrows), consistent with an acute DVT. Contrast outlining the thrombus produces the characteristic "tram-track" appearance.

of acute lower extremity DVT. Findings include discrete-filling defects outlined by contrast in the vein ("tram-track" sign) or an abrupt cutoff in the column of contrast. Contrast-enhanced CT can detect DVT in the larger central veins (iliacs, IVC), which appear as low-attenuation thrombus within the vein with peripheral enhancement. Extrinsic compression of the veins by pelvic or abdominal masses can also easily be seen with CT. Magnetic resonance venography has a greater than 85% accuracy for detecting DVT. Thrombi appear as either a venous segment without flow signal or as a discrete intralumi-nal-filling defect on TOF imaging. The thrombus may appear dark or bright on TOF imaging, depending on the age of the thrombus.

With the widespread use of central venous catheters, the incidence of upper extremity DVT has increased. Once thought to be benign, it is now estimated that approximately 15% of pulmonary emboli originate from the upper extremities. Fortunately, the incidence of fatal pulmonary emboli is less from the upper extremities than it is from the lower extremities. Patients may be asymptomatic or present with arm or face swelling, or both. The modalities used to diagnose upper extremity DVT are similar to those for lower extremity DVT, including duplex ultrasound, venography, contrast-enhanced CT, and magnetic resonance venography. Anticoagulation therapy with heparin is the treatment of choice; thrombolysis is reserved for symptomatic cases.

SELECTED REFERENCES

Lynch TG, Dalsing MC, Ouriel K, et al. Developments in diagnosis and classification of venous disorders: non-invasive diagnosis. Cardiovasc Surg. 1999; 7: 160–178.

Carretta RF. Scintigraphic imaging of lower-extremity acute venous thrombosis. Adv Ther. 1998; 15: 315–322.

Gottlieb RH, Widjaja J, Mehra S, Robinette WB. Clinical outcomes of untreated symptomatic patients with negative findings on sonography of the thigh for deep vein thrombosis: our experience and a review of the literature. AJR. 1999; 172: 1601–1604.

Fraser JD, Anderson DR. Deep venous thrombosis: recent advances and optimal investigation with US. Radiology. 1999; 211: 9–24.

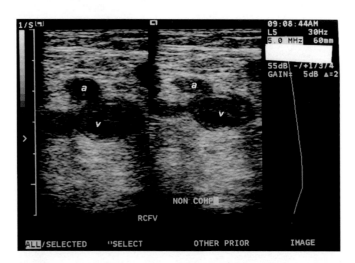

Figure 5–5 Acute deep venous thrombosis. Duplex sonography of the common femoral vein in a patient with acute leg swelling. Echogenic thrombus is seen within the noncompressible vein (**v** represents vein; **a**, artery).

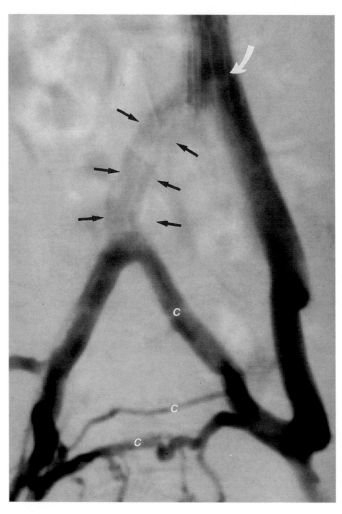

Figure 5–6 Chronic deep venous thrombosis (DVT). A pelvic venogram in a patient with longstanding DVT shows multiple thin, linear-filling defects and diminished opacification of the recanalized right common iliac vein (arrows). Multiple venous collaterals are present (**c**) that drain into the left iliac vein. A previously inserted IVC filter has caudally migrated and is positioned at the confluence of the iliac veins (curved arrow).

5.3 EFFORT THROMBOSIS (PAGET-SCHROETTER SYNDROME)

Effort thrombosis of the upper extremity, also known as Paget-Schroetter syndrome or primary axillosubclavian vein thrombosis, is a form of posttraumatic thrombosis of the axillary vein caused by extrinsic compression of the axillary vein by the scalenus muscle or by the costocoracoid ligament during forced abduction. It is usually seen in younger individuals following strenuous exercise or activity. Depending on the extent of venous thrombosis and the degree of collateral venous drainage, some patients may be asymptomatic, whereas others experience symptoms of venous hypertension (arm swelling and heaviness).

Less symptomatic patients may be placed on anticoagulation therapy alone; more symptomatic patients should undergo catheter-directed thrombolysis. Once the clot burden has been cleared, a venogram will show impingement or occlusion of the axillary vein. The finding of venous compression may be augmented by performing venography during provocative maneuvers. These include hyperabduction-external rotation of the arm, deep inspiration with the head facing the unaffected side (Adson's maneuver), or external rotation of the scapula (costoclavicular maneuver). Although ultrasound and magnetic resonance venography have been used for diagnosing thrombotic central venous occlusion, provocative maneuvers are more difficult, and the etiology of the venous obstruction may not be identified.

If venous compression is proven, definitive therapy using transaxillary 1st rib resection is recommended.

SELECTED REFERENCES

Machleder HI. Thrombolytic therapy and surgery for primary axillosubclavian vein thrombosis: current approach. Semin Vasc Surg. 1996; 9: 46–49.

Kunkel JM, Machleder HI. Spontaneous subclavian vein thrombosis: a successful combined approach of local thrombolytic therapy followed by first rib resection. Surgery. 1989; 106: 114.

Sheeran SR, Hallisey MJ, Murphy TP, et al. Local thrombolytic therapy as part of a multidisciplinary approach to acute axillosubclavian vein thrombosis (Paget-Schroetter syndrome). J Vasc Interv Radiol. 1997; 8: 253–260.

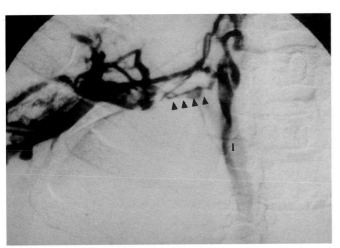

A

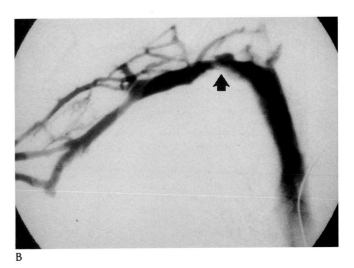

B

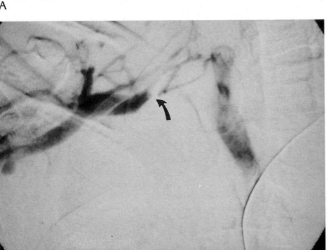

C

Figure 5–7A–C Effort thrombosis (Paget-Schroetter syndrome). A right subclavian venogram (**A**) shows thrombosis of the right subclavian vein (arrowheads) with collateral reconstitution of the innominate vein (**I**). The patient was a young female student who frequently carried a heavy bookbag with her right arm and shoulder. After catheter-directed thrombolytic therapy and venous angioplasty, there is restored patency of the subclavian vein (**B**). A residual stenosis due to chronic impingement and thickening of the caudal aspect of the vein is noted (arrow). A venogram obtained with the right arm hyperabducted and externally rotated (**C**) shows characteristic compression and occlusion of the subclavian vein in the costoclavicular space (curved arrow). The patient subsequently underwent transaxillary resection of the first rib.

5.4 PERIPHERAL ARTERIAL OCCLUSIVE DISEASE

Peripheral vascular disease (PVD) is most commonly due to atherosclerosis and is an age-dependent condition. Recognized risk factors include smoking, hypertension, diabetes, hyperlipidemia, obesity, atherosclerotic cardiovascular disease, and a family history of arteriosclerosis. Disease severity is categorized according to three distinct grades: claudication (grade 1), rest pain (grade 2), and ischemic ulceration or tissue loss (grade 3). Nearly 70% of patients with chronic peripheral arterial occlusive disease will have a stable pattern of disease, and an additional 15% will experience modest improvements in symptomatology with exercise and medical therapy alone. The mechanism of the vascular benefits of exercise are uncertain, but appear to be mediated in part through altered muscle metabolism, improved red blood cell rheology, and changes in microcirculatory flow. Recent data with cilostazol and clopidogrel have also shown these medications to be effective in preventing the clinical progression of disease.

Acute lower limb ischemia (ALLI) may occur secondary to embolic occlusion or thrombosis of a previously diseased vessel. Clinically, this condition is manifested by the six "p's": pain, pallor, pulselessness, paralysis, paresthesia, and poikilothermia (coldness). The severity of symptoms and response to attempted revascularization directly correlates with the extent of vascular involvement and the status of adjacent arterial collaterals. Digital subtraction angiography will show the level and length of the occlusion, the patency of collaterals, and the condition of the tibial vessels, all of which are prognostic of the immediate and long-term benefits of revascularization. Definitive surgical or percutaneous therapy should be instituted as early as possible because ongoing ischemia may result in mus-

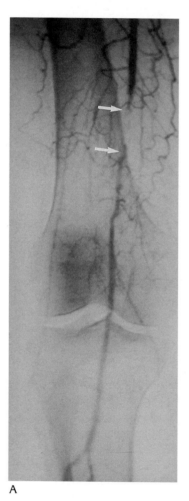

A

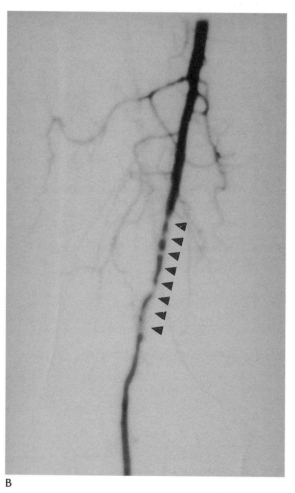

B

Figure 5–8A–D Peripheral arterial occlusion. Arteriography of the right leg (**A**) shows a short occlusion of the superficial femoral artery (SFA) at the level of the adductor canal (arrows), a common location for femoral atherosclerosis. Numerous collaterals suggest the presence of a chronic underlying stenosis. After thrombolytic therapy (**B**), there is restored arterial patency revealing tandem high-grade SFA and popliteal stenoses (arrowheads). This was treated with balloon angioplasty (**C**) with resolution of the stenosis (**D**). The margins of the initial occlusion are marked with arrows.

cle necrosis and compartment syndromes. Several large studies have evaluated the role of thrombolytic therapy and surgical thrombectomy in patients with ALLI. For patients with acute (<7 days) symptoms, an absence of profound ischemia, and no contraindications, percutaneous catheter-directed thrombolytic therapy allows limb salvage in most cases and reduces the incidence of cardiovascular mortality as compared with surgical thrombectomy. Improved clinical success correlates with a short duration of occlusion, limited length of arterial involvement, the ability to cross the occluded segment with a guidewire, adequate patent distal arterial runoff, and the presence of a treatable underlying stenosis. Longer duration (>2 weeks) occlusions and patients with profound ischemia should be initially treated by surgical thrombectomy or bypass.

SELECTED REFERENCES

Palfreyman SJ, Michaels JA. Vascular surgical society of Great Britain and Ireland: systematic review of intra-arterial thrombolytic therapy for peripheral vascular occlusions. Br J Surg. 1999; 86: 704.

Weaver FA, Comerota AJ, Youngblood M, et al. Surgical revascularization versus thrombolysis for nonembolic lower extremity native artery occlusions: results of a prospective randomized trial. The STILE Investigators. Surgery versus Thrombolysis for Ischemia of the Lower Extremity. J Vasc Surg. 1996; 24: 513–521.

Ouriel K, Veith FJ, Sasahara AA. A comparison of recombinant urokinase with vascular surgery as initial treatment for acute arterial occlusion of the legs. Thrombolysis or Peripheral Arterial Surgery (TOPAS) Investigators. N Engl J Med. 1998; 338: 1105–1111.

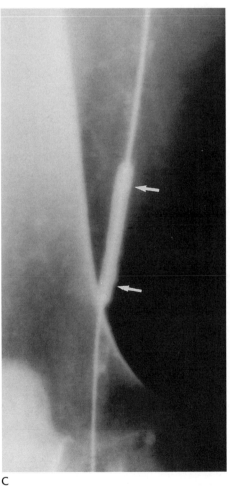

C

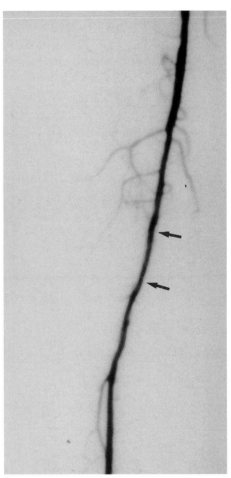

D

5.5 POPLITEAL ARTERY ANEURYSM

Popliteal artery aneurysms (defined as >50% enlargement of the popliteal artery compared with the distal SFA) are the most common peripheral aneurysms, and may be isolated or occur as part of the arteria magna syndrome. This latter condition occurs in older men, is not directly related to smoking or other cardiovascular risk factors, and is histologically unique with disruption of the normal arterial media and elastica. Patients with arteria magna syndrome have diffuse lower extremity arterial dilation and elongation, sluggish antegrade flow, and arterial aneurysms in three quarters of cases.

Popliteal aneurysms affect a younger population than most patients with atherosclerosis, are most commonly located just distal to the adductor hiatus, and are associated with multiple aneurysms in other sites, including the abdominal aorta. In younger patients with peripheral vascular disease as well as in older patients presenting with the blue-toe syndrome and a palpable mass in the popliteal fossa, duplex ultrasound or computed tomography is often the first test and can often reliably reveal the presence of an aneurysm. Since aneurysms may be bilateral in up to 58% of cases, an evaluation of the asymptomatic limb is also necessary. Once identified, popliteal aneurysms require prompt surgical repair due to an otherwise high risk of acute thrombosis, distal embolization, and limb loss. Preoperative angiography should be performed to provide an evaluation of the extent of arterial involvement and the patency of the tibial runoff vessels for supporting a distal bypass. On occasion, thrombolytic therapy may be used to uncover the presence of a popliteal aneurysm in a patient presenting with an occluded popliteal artery of uncertain origin, and to restore the patency of embolically occluded distal vessels prior to surgery.

SELECTED REFERENCES

Shortell CK, DeWeese JA, Ouriel K, et al. Popliteal artery aneurysms: a 25-year surgical experience. J Vasc Surg. 1991; 13: 398.

Rizzo RJ, Flinn WR, Yao JST, et al. Computed tomography for evaluation of arterial disease in the popliteal fossa. J Vasc Surg. 1990; 11: 112.

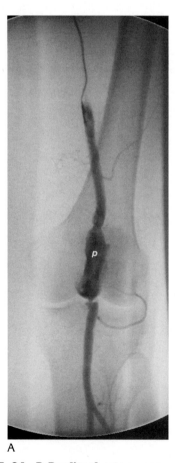

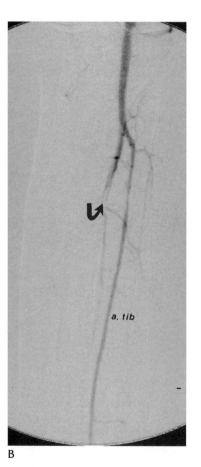

A

B

Figure 5–9A, B Popliteal artery aneurysm. A left popliteal arteriogram in a patient with blue-toe syndrome identifies aneurysmal enlargement (**p**) of the popliteal artery behind the knee (**A**). Imaging of the arterial runoff (**B**) shows embolic occlusion of the tibioperoneal trunk (curved arrow) due to thrombus dislodged from the aneurysm. The anterior tibial artery (**a. tib**) remains patent. The patient was treated with thrombolytic therapy.

5.6 POPLITEAL ENTRAPMENT

In young patients presenting with claudication or acute ischemia of the legs, possible causative considerations include a popliteal mass (eg, Baker's cyst), popliteal artery aneurysm, cystic adventitial disease, embolic occlusion, and popliteal entrapment. Popliteal entrapment is more common in men, and may be bilateral in up to two thirds of cases. Five types have been described on the basis of the relationship of the artery to the gastrocnemius muscle insertion or popliteus muscle tendon.

Both magnetic resonance imaging and ultrasonography may be used to reveal the abnormal soft tissue structures compressing the artery although MRI is preferred modality because it provides superior anatomic depiction. Angiography will show the characteristic medial deviation of the popliteal artery, which is accentuated by passive dorsiflexion or forced plantar flexion of the foot. Associated angiographic findings include arterial irregularity from chronic repetitive trauma, focal arterial dilatation, popliteal occlusion, and distal embolic disease. Recent experience with CT arteriography has also shown promise for detecting both the vascular abnormalities and the cause of arterial compression. Treatment consists of surgical release of the artery, and early repair is associated with an improved long-term functional outcome.

SELECTED REFERENCES

Ring DH Jr, Haines GA, Miller DL. Popliteal artery entrapment syndrome: arteriographic findings and thrombolytic therapy. J Vasc Interv Radiol. 1999; 10: 713–721.

Atilla S, Akpek ET, Yucel C, et al. MR imaging and MR angiography in popliteal artery entrapment syndrome. Eur Radiol. 1998; 8: 1025–1029.

Marzo L, Cavallaro A, Mingoli A, et al. Popliteal artery entrapment syndrome: the role of early diagnosis and treatment. Surgery. 1997; 122: 26–31.

MacSweeney S, Cuming R, Greenhalgh RM. Colour Doppler ultrasonographic imaging in the diagnosis of popliteal artery entrapment syndrome. Br J Surg. 1995; 82: 569–570.

Beregi JP, Djabbari M, Desmoucelle F, et al. Popliteal vascular disease: evaluation with spiral CT angiography. Radiology. 1997; 203: 477–483.

Guerra J, Lee BY. Popliteal artery entrapment syndrome. Contemp Surg. 1995; 4: 6–10.

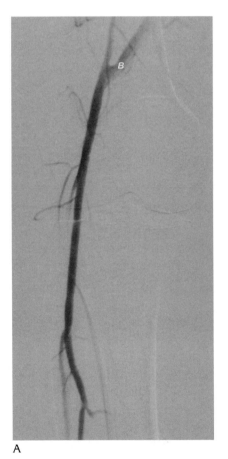
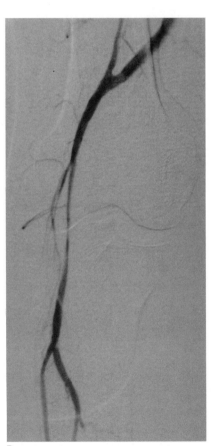

A   B

Figure 5–10A, B Popliteal entrapment. An arteriogram obtained with the leg in the neutral position shows a normal popliteal artery (**A**). The patient has had a prior femoral-to-above-knee popliteal bypass (**B**). After forced plantar-flexion (**B**), there is smooth concentric narrowing and mild medial displacement of the popliteal artery.

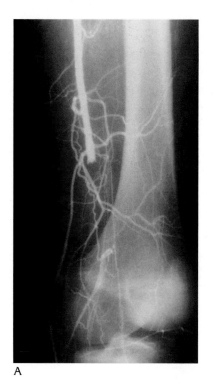

A

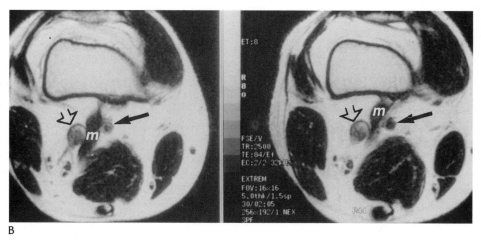

B

Figure 5–11A–C Popliteal entrapment. Arteriography shows occlusion of the proximal popliteal artery (**A**). An MRI on the same patient (**B**) reveals a type IV popliteal entrapment, with compression on the artery by an abnormally inserting popliteal muscle (**m**). (open arrow represents vein; straight arrow, artery). A line drawing shows the normal relationships of the popliteal artery, veins, and muscles (**C**). The popliteal muscle is anterior to the vessels.

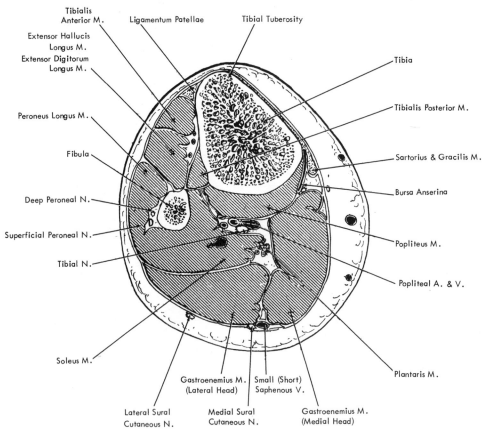

C

5.7 THORACIC OUTLET SYNDROME

As they exit the thorax, the subclavian vessels and brachial plexus course through three sites of potential extrinsic compression: the interscalene triangle, formed by the anterior and medial scalene muscles and the first rib (most common type); the costoclavicular space, formed by the clavicle and subclavius muscle superiorly and the first rib inferiorly, and the pectoralis minor tunnel, formed by the pectoralis minor tendon and the coracoid process. Neurologic involvement (pain, tingling, numbness) is most common. Other symptoms include Raynaud's phenomenon (40%), arm swelling, venous thrombosis, decreased skin temperature, intermittent claudication, and ischemia or cyanosis of the digits.

When the diagnosis of thoracic outlet syndrome is entertained, a chest radiograph should be reviewed for the presence of a cervical rib, an occasionally associated finding. Upper extremity venography of the affected limb may appear normal or may show narrowing or irregularity of the subclavian vein at the junction of the clavicle and first rib. If the venogram is normal with the arm in the neutral position, the study should be repeated with the arm abducted and the head rotated toward the unaffected side; a positive study will show the resulting impingement of the superior aspect of the subclavian vein as it passes over the first rib. When the artery is affected, angiographic findings include mild dilatation or frank aneurysmal enlargement of the distal subclavian artery (the most common finding), arterial displacement, focal stenosis, and distal embolization. Provocative maneuvers (eg, abduction of the arm) can be used to facilitate the diagnosis, although more than 30% of normal people can have abnormal findings after these maneuvers. Recently, magnetic resonance angiography has been used to successfully show vascular impingement, allowing simultaneous visualization of neural involvement and associated soft tissue anomalies.

SELECTED REFERENCES

McCarthy MJ, Varty K, London NJ, Bell PR. Experience of supraclavicular exploration and decompression for treatment of thoracic outlet syndrome. Ann Vasc Surg. 1999; 13: 268–274.

Abe M, Ichinohe K, Nishida J. Diagnosis, treatment, and complications of thoracic outlet syndrome. J Orthop Sci. 1999; 4: 66–69.

Redenbach DM, Nelems B. A comparative study of structures comprising the thoracic outlet in 250 human cadavers and 72 surgical cases of thoracic outlet syndrome. Eur J Cardiothorac Surg. 1998; 13: 353–360.

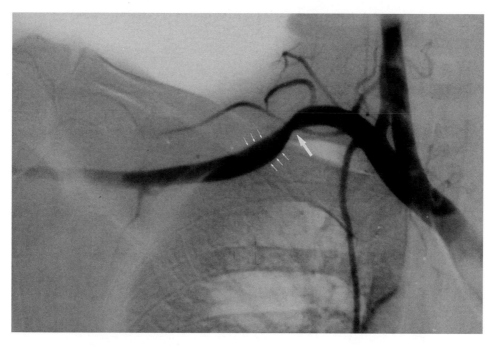

Figure 5–12 Thoracic outlet syndrome. A right subclavian arteriogram shows a chronic focal stenosis (large arrow) in the location of the anterior scalene muscle. Mild poststenotic dilatation is present (small arrows).

5.8 HYPOTHENAR HAMMER SYNDROME

Hypothenar hammer syndrome occurs as a result of repetitive trauma to the ulnar artery as it passes over the hamate bone, and is thus seen in people who regularly use their palms for pushing, pounding, or hammering (jackhammer operators, farmers, martial artists, and professional athletes who use a racket or bat). This results in spasm and thrombosis of the smaller vessels of the distal palmar arch and metacarpals, and in pseudoaneurysm formation in the larger arteries of the proximal palmar arch. Thrombus developing within these pseudoaneurysms may cause distal embolization with consequent ischemia and necrosis of the digits. Clinically, patients present with digital ischemia, Raynaud's phenomenon, or a pulsatile mass on the hypothenar eminence. Symptoms are often aggravated by exposure to cold. Arteriography is the gold standard for making the diagnosis, and may show spasm or irregularity of the ulnar artery in a characteristic location over the hypothenar eminence, pseudoaneurysm formation, or embolic occlusion of the digital arteries.

SELECTED REFERENCES

Van de Walle PM, Moll FL, De Smet AA. The hypothenar hammer syndrome: update and literature review. Acta Chir Belg. 1998; 98: 116–119.

Wheatley MJ, Marx MV. The use of intra-arterial urokinase in the management of hand ischemia secondary to palmar and digital arterial occlusion. Ann Plast Surg. 1996; 37: 356–362.

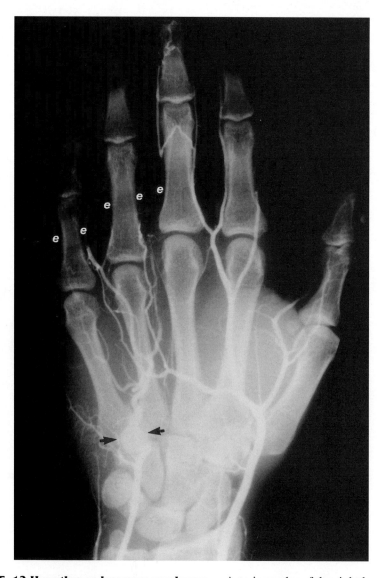

Figure 5–13 Hypothenar hammer syndrome. Arteriography of the right hand shows a focal pseudoaneurysm of the ulnar artery just beneath the hypothenar eminence (black arrows). There is thrombosis of the superficial palmar arch and embolic occlusion (**e**) of multiple digital arteries on the medial aspect of the hand.

5.9 FEMORAL PSEUDOANEURYSM AND ARTERIOVENOUS FISTULA

Femoral artery complications, including femoral arteriovenous fistulas and pseudoaneurysms, occur in less than 1% of peripheral catheterizations. As the number of percutaneous vascular procedures has increased, so has the recognition of femoral artery complications.

Femoral arteriovenous fistulas (AVFs) occur when the femoral vein is traversed while puncturing the femoral artery. A branch of the profunda femoral artery is commonly involved. AVFs may be clinically silent or present as a bruit in the groin, leg swelling, worsening varicosities, leg ischemia, or congestive heart failure. In symptomatic cases, the diagnosis is confirmed

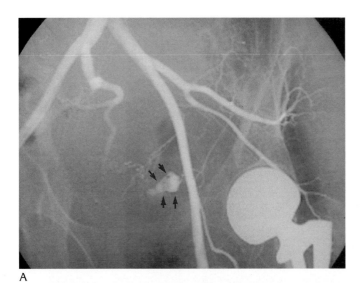

A

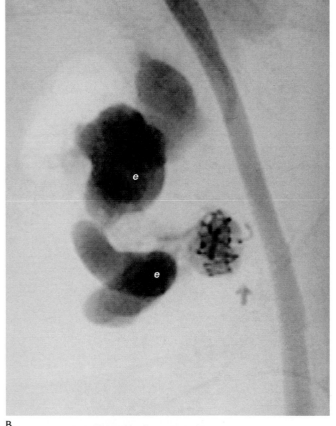

B

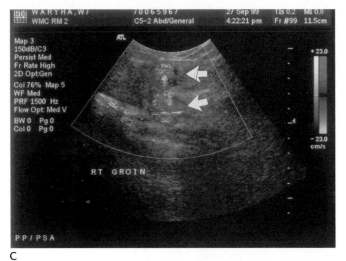

C

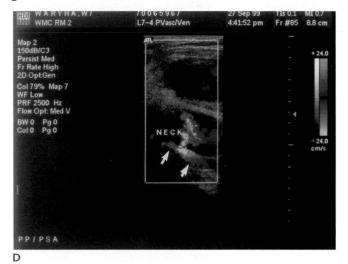

D

Figure 5–14A–D Femoral pseudoaneurysm. An iliac arteriogram in the left anterior oblique projection (**A**) shows an extraluminal collection of contrast (arrows) at the site of a previous high femoral catheterization. After selective cannulation and coil embolization (**B**), there is nearly complete occlusion of the pseudoaneurysm. Contrast seen medial to the pseudoaneurysm represents retroperitoneal extravasation (**e**) from the initial arteriogram. Color-flow Doppler imaging of a different patient (**C, D**) shows a bilobed pseudoaneurysm (**C**, large arrows) arising from the common femoral artery (**D**, small arrows). There is a narrow neck at the base of the pseudoaneurysm.

by Doppler ultrasonography. Sonography will show pulsatile arterial flow in the region of the fistula, and retrograde flow and/or abnormally high spectral velocities will be seen within the involved vein. Occasionally, the fistulous tract may be directly visualized. Angiography shows early filling of the veins and usually displays the fistula.

Femoral pseudoaneurysms usually develop after catheter removal, and represent contained arterial leaking from the puncture site. Doppler ultrasound is again the noninvasive diagnostic modality of choice, revealing contained extravascular blood flow. In addition, simultaneous ultrasound-guided compression at the site of leakage can often successfully resolve the pseudoaneurysm. More recently, the ultrasound-guided percutaneous injection of thrombin has been used to occlude femoral pseudoaneurysms. Angiographically, pseudoaneurysms appear as extravascular collections of contrast, which fill from the injured artery.

SELECTED REFERENCES

Chatterjee T, Do DD, Mahler F, Meier B. A prospective, randomized evaluation of nonsurgical closure of femoral pseudoaneurysm by compression device with or without ultrasound guidance. Catheter Cardiovasc Interv. 1999; 47: 304–309.

Ruebben A, Tettoni S, Muratore P, et al. Arteriovenous fistulas induced by femoral arterial catheterization: percutaneous treatment. Radiology. 1998; 209: 729–734.

Kumins NH, Landau DS, Montalvo J, et al. Expanded indications for the treatment of postcatheterization femoral pseudoaneurysms with ultrasound-guided compression. Am J Surg. 1998; 176: 131–136.

Lee BY, Madden JL, Hershman A. Femoral arteriovenous fistula. Am J Surg. 1970; 120: 390–392.

Lee BY, Trainer FS. Regional hemodynamics of arteriovenous fistula. In: *Peripheral Vascular Surgery: Hemodynamics of Arterial Pulsatile Blood Flow.* New York, NY: Appleton-Century-Crofts; 1973: 160–181.

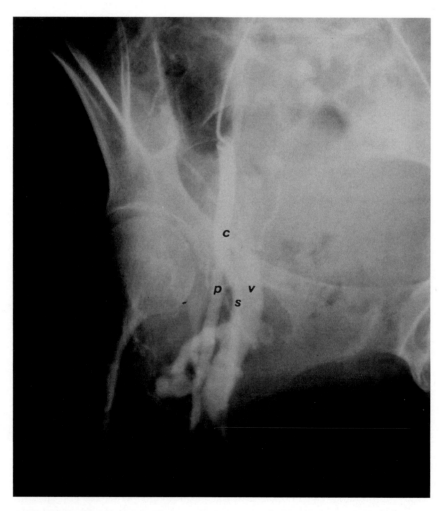

Figure 5–15 Femoral arteriovenous fistula. Right femoral arteriography shows simultaneous filling of the artery and vein in the right groin. The patient had recent transfemoral cardiac catheterization. (**c** represents common femoral artery; **p**, profunda femoral artery; **s**, superficial femoral artery; **v**, common femoral vein).

5.10 TRAUMATIC ARTERIAL INJURY

Blunt or penetrating trauma may result in several types of vascular damage. Potential injuries include pseudoaneurysm formation, transection, intimal laceration or intramural hematoma (dissection type injuries), arteriovenous fistulas, or spasm. The nature of the trauma, physical examination, and site of trauma indicate the necessity for diagnostic evaluation and the type of imaging that should be performed. Plain radiographs of the affected site are insensitive to the presence of arterial disruption. Computed tomography will identify any hemorrhage adjacent to the injured vessel, and may show a traumatic dissection or pseudoaneurysm in larger vessels. Angiography remains the diagnostic modality of choice, and is indicated for patients with objective clinical findings of potential vascular injury and for patients with asymptomatic proximity injuries of the neck, thoracic outlet, abdomen, and extremities. In such patients, an angiographic abnormality will be detected in 1–12%. Patients sustaining a posterior knee dislocation should also be considered for angiographic evaluation due to an approximately 30% incidence of associated popliteal artery injury and consequent high risk for limb loss if untreated. Minimal injuries (no active bleeding or obstruction to arterial blood flow) have an unpredictable natural history and a reported incidence of symptomatic progression ranging from 9–50%. However, close clinical follow-up is generally sufficient; operative or transcatheter intervention can be performed in the event of clinical deterioration.

Many injuries identified by angiography are amenable to simultaneous transcatheter treatment. Small extravasating vessels can be occluded using transcatheter embolization, and flow-limiting dissection may be treatable by prolonged angioplasty or placement of an intravascular stent to tack down the obstructing lesion. The recent development and clinical application of stent-supported grafts offers a promising, less invasive treatment option for patients with major vascular injury.

SELECTED REFERENCES

Dennis JW, Frykberg ER, Veldenz HC, et al. Validation of nonoperative management of occult vascular injuries and accuracy of physical examination alone in penetrating extremity trauma: 5-to 10-year follow-up. J Trauma 1998; 44: 243–252.

Hoffer EK, Sclafani SJ, Herskowitz MM, Scalea TM. Natural history of arterial injuries diagnosed with arteriography. J Vasc Interv Radiol. 1997; 6(1 pt 1): 43–53.

Frykberg ER, Crump JM, Dennis JW, et al. Nonoperative observation of clinically occult arterial injuries: a prospective evaluation. Surgery. 1991; 109: 85–96.

Kaufman SL, Martin LG. Arterial injuries associated with complete dislocation of the knee. Radiology. 1992; 109: 153–155.

Gaskill-Shipley MF, Tomsick TA. Exploratory and interventional angiography in severe trauma: present and future procedure of choice. Radiographics. 1996; 6: 963–970.

Figure 5–16 Traumatic vascular injury. A left brachial arteriogram of a patient suffering from a gunshot wound to the arm and chest shows an incomplete transection and traumatic pseudoaneurysm (arrowheads) at the site of arterial injury. The associated intimal injury is evident as a linear-filling defect on the lateral side of the artery (small arrows). A bullet fragment is retained in the chest wall (**B**). Arterial injuries such as these may be caused by transmitted forces from a proximity wound rather than by direct vessel trauma.

5.11 POSTERIOR KNEE DISLOCATION

Posterior knee dislocations are usually a sequela of an automobile accident in which the impact of the knee against the dashboard of the car displaces the femur posteriorly relative to the tibia. Popliteal artery injury occurs in approximately 30–40% of posterior knee dislocations, and is the result of stretching or transection of the artery at its muscularly fixed position behind the knee joint. Because of a very high rate of limb loss, it was once recommended (and is still endorsed by many) that angiography be performed for all patients sustaining this injury. Current practice, however, advocates close observation, with angiography performed only in those patients with ischemia, a weakened pulse, or an ipsilaterally cooler foot. In affected patients, angiography can show many findings, including active extravasation, intimal injury, pseudoaneurysm formation, arteriovenous fistula formation, and complete occlusion. Sonography of the popliteal fossa has also been suggested as the initial test for patients with a suspected arterial injury. Acute thrombosis can be detected on ultrasound as echogenic material within the vessel lumen and intimal injuries may be seen as mural irregularity. An ultrasound screening examination of the popliteal artery, such as the FAST examination of the abdomen, may in the future become the screening test of choice.

SELECTED REFERENCES

Wascher DC, Dvirnak PC, DeCoster TA. Knee dislocation: initial assessment and implications for treatment. J Orthop Trauma. 1997; 11: 525–529.

Jones RE, Smith EC, Bone GE. Vascular and orthopedic complications of knee dislocation. Surg Gynecol Obstet. 1979; 149: 554–558.

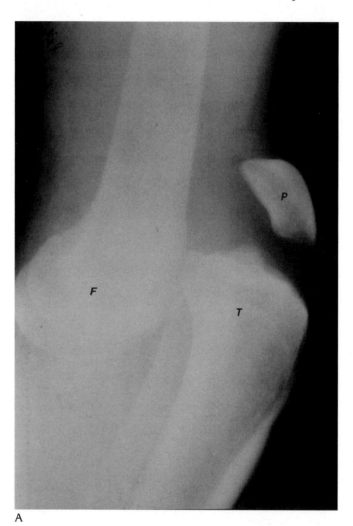

A

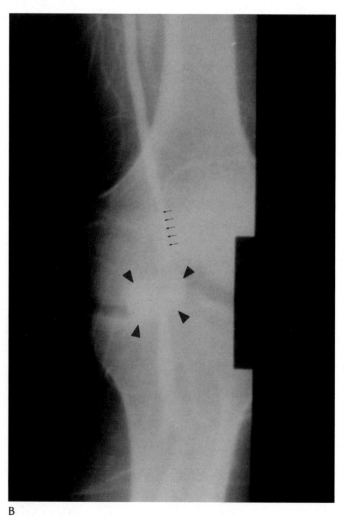

B

Figure 5–17A, B Posterior knee dislocation. A lateral radiograph of the knee (**A**) reveals a posterior dislocation of the femur (**F**) with respect to the tibia (**T**) and patella (**P**). After knee reduction, an AP arteriogram (**B**) shows an intimal tear (small arrows) and pseudoaneurysm (arrowheads) of the popliteal artery due to traumatic shearing and stretching of the vessel.

5.12 ELBOW FRACTURE/DISLOCATION

Up to 7% of patients with traumatic elbow dislocations incur an injury to the brachial artery, usually due to stretching of the vessel. Initially absent pulses may return after elbow reduction, and further imaging in these cases is often not warranted. However, for patients with a persistent pulse deficit or expanding hematoma, immediate angiography should be performed. This may show compression and displacement of the brachial artery by osseous and soft tissue structures and hematoma. Intimal disruption with luminal irregularity can be noted. Arterial occlusions may be secondary to an obstructive intimal flap or arterial avulsion, although numerous collaterals usually prevent the development of severe ischemia. In cases with an associated fracture, laceration of the artery causing a pseudoaneurysm or active contrast extravasation dictates the need for urgent surgical exploration.

SELECTED REFERENCES

Platz A, Heinzelmann M, Ertel W, Trentz O. Posterior elbow dislocation with associated vascular injury after blunt trauma. J Trauma. 1999; 46: 948–950.

Endean ED, Veldenz HC, Schwarcz TH, Hyde GL. Recognition of arterial injury in elbow dislocation. J Vasc Surg. 1992; 16: 402–406.

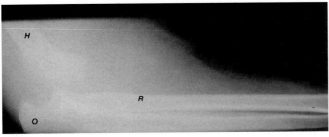

A

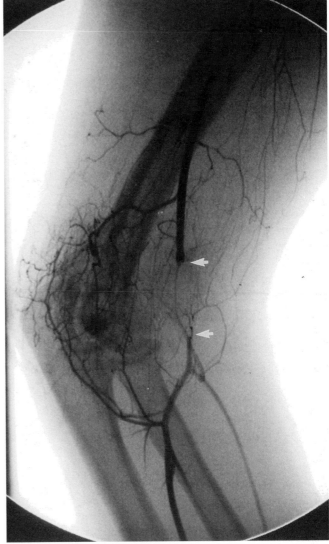

B

Figure 5–18A, B Elbow dislocation. A lateral radiograph of the elbow (**A**) shows posterior dislocation of the ulnar-humeral joint (**H** represents humerus; **O**, olecranon process of the ulna; **R**, radius). On an angiogram performed after elbow reduction (**B**), there is traumatic occlusion of the distal brachial artery (arrows). In addition, the artery is lifted away from the bone due to an adjacent hematoma.

CHAPTER 6

CATHETERS AND TUBES

Maurice R. Poplausky, MD

John H. Rundback, MD

Bok Y. Lee, MD, FACS

6.1 CENTRAL VENOUS CATHETERS

Central venous catheters (CVC) are frequently used to provide hemodynamic monitoring, parenteral medications, total parenteral nutrition, fluid resuscitation, and dialysis access. Catheters are available in a wide variety of sizes, and may have 1, 2, or 3 lumens. Types of devices include short-term non-tunneled, intermediate-term tunneled, and long-term subcutaneously inserted ports. Both the subclavian and internal jugular vein access sites may be used, although the subclavian site is associated with a higher incidence of both pneumothorax and venous thrombosis. While generally safe, complications do occur from CVC insertion. Potential complications include in-fection, catheter malpositioning, catheter occlusion, pneumothorax, hemothorax, arterial injury, and catheter fracture. Chest radiographs are generally adequate for evaluating the position of centrally placed catheters and for recognizing associated complications. Catheters should follow the expected venous course, with the tip positioned at the right heart border (right atrium). The presence of a pneumothorax should be searched for diligently in any patient where an attempt at central venous access was made. If catheter location is still a question after review of the chest radiograph, contrast injection into the catheter under fluoroscopy will reveal its precise location.

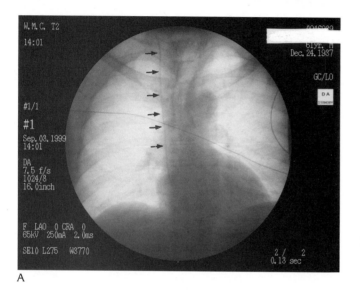

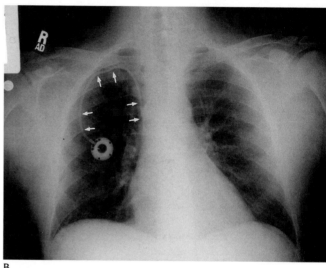

A

B

Figure 6–1A, B Central venous catheters.   Normal right internal jugular triple-lumen catheter (**A**) and right subclavian venous port (SVP, **B**). In each case, the catheter is marked with arrows and the catheter tip is positioned in the right atrium.

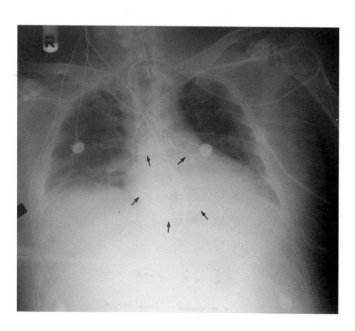

Figure 6–2 Normal Swan-Ganz catheter.   The tip of the catheter is located within the right main pulmonary artery. With balloon inflation, the catheter wedges into a segmental branch.

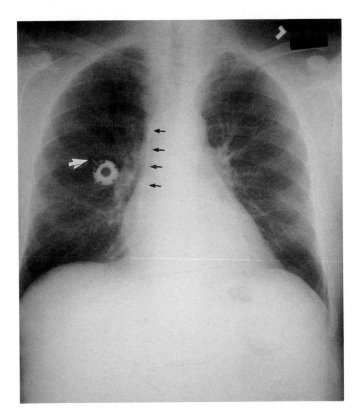

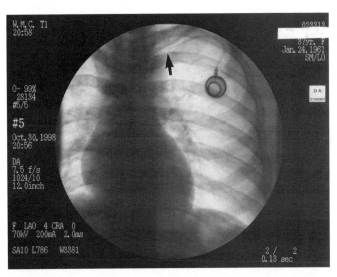

Figure 6–4 "Pinch-off" syndrome. There is a subclavian single-lumen port on the left side. The catheter is fractured at the junction of the clavicle and first rib (arrow). The distal catheter fragment has been percutaneously retrieved from the pulmonary artery.

Figure 6–3 Disconnected titanium port. The single-lumen port reservoir is seen over the right chest wall. The catheter has dislodged from the port attachment (white arrow) and is located within the superior vena cava and right atrium (black arrows).

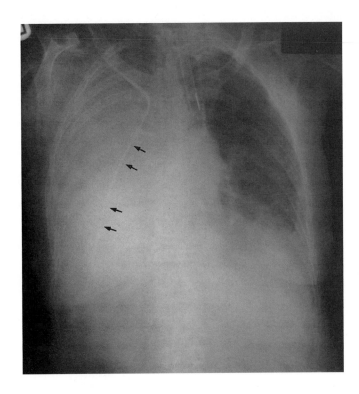

Figure 6–5 Misplaced central venous catheter in pleural space. The tip of the catheter is within the right hemithorax (arrows). Administered saline causes extensive opacification on the right side.

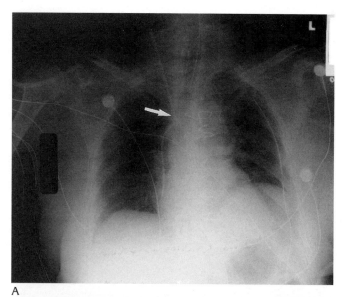

A

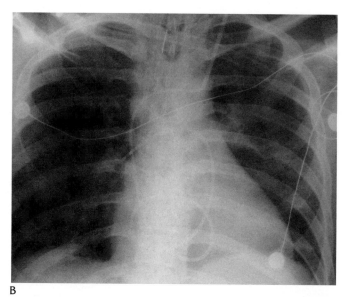

B

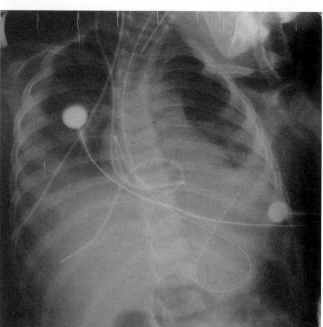

C

Figure 6–6A–C Knotted and coiled Swan-Ganz catheters.
A knot is seen within the subclavian venous catheter (**A,** arrow). Catheter coiling is seen within the right atrium and ventricle (**B, C**). The tip of the catheter (in **C**) is in the right hepatic vein.

Figure 6–7A, B Central venous catheter arterial misplacement. The course of a right-sided catheter (**A**) is consistent with intra-arterial placement through the innominate artery and aortic arch (arrows). (**B**) Contrast injection shows the tip to be in the aorta (**Ao**).

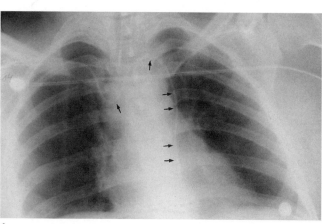

A

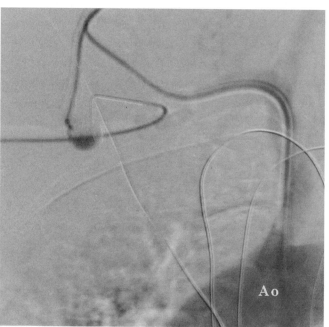

B

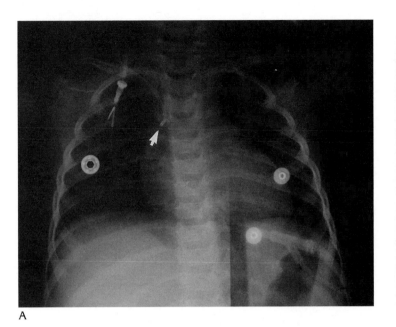
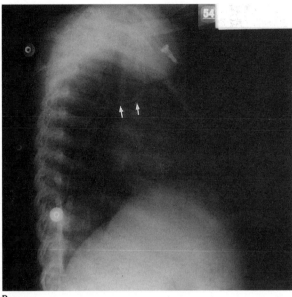

A

B

Figure 6–8A, B Catheter in azygous vein. AP (**A**) and lateral (**B**) radiographs of the chest show the tip of the central venous catheter to point posteriorly into the azygous vein (arrows).

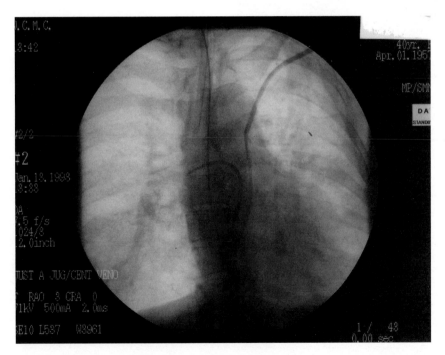

Figure 6–9 Catheter in left-sided superior vena cava. An AP chest film shows a left subclavian Swan-Ganz catheter traversing a left-sided superior vena cava, coronary sinus, right atrium, right ventricle, and pulmonary artery.

6.2 CHEST TUBES

Surgically or percutaneously placed chest tubes are frequently inserted postoperatively, and are also indicated for the treatment of pneumothorax, hemothorax, empyema, large pleural effusions, and for transcatheter pleurodesis. Surgical tubes are usually placed in the 4th intercostal space in the midclavicular line. Although smaller tubes are generally acceptable for evacuating the pleural air causing a pneumothorax, large air leaks may require the insertion of a larger bore tube. For drainages other than loculated collections, the tube should lie posterior to the lung and be directed at the lung apex. For pneumothoraces, the tube should lie anterior to the lung, also directed toward the apex of the lung. The chest tube itself is radiopaque and has a linear radiopaque marker on it. There is a "break" in the linear marker, indicating the location of the sideholes. The sideholes of the tube must be within the pleural space to maintain function and avoid subcutaneous emphysema. Chest radiographs are usually adequate to evaluate chest tube position. CT scans are excellent for evaluating the position of chest tubes when questions arise. Complications of tube placement include bleeding, pulmonary injury or damage to adjacent organs (eg, liver, heart, vessels).

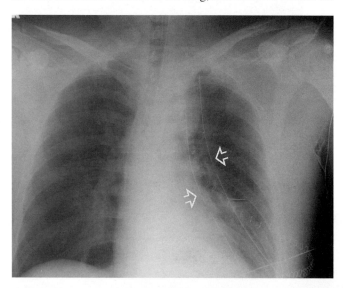

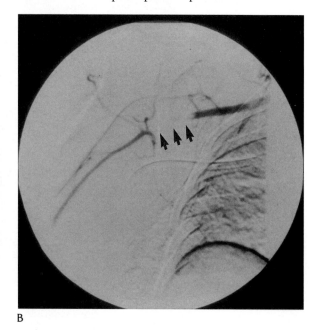

Figure 6–10 Normal chest tubes. The normal position of anterior and posterior chest tubes (open arrows) in the left hemithorax is noted in a post-operative patient.

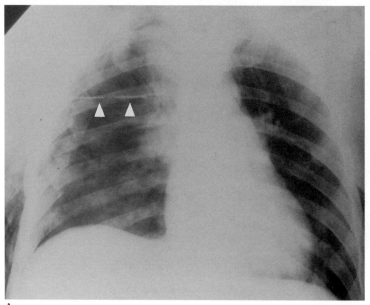

A

B

Figure 6–11A, B Axillary artery injury from chest tube insertion. A PA chest radiograph shows a right-sided chest tube to be overlying the upper hemithorax (**A**, arrowheads). An upper extremity arteriogram on the same patient (**B**) reveals an occlusion of the axillary artery (black arrows) due to a traumatic injury occurring at the time of tube placement.

6.3 NASOGASTRIC TUBES

Nasogastric tubes(NGT) and nasojejunal tubes are used for gastric decompression, administration of tube feedings, gastric lavage, and prior to performing small bowel contrast studies. Various caliber and length tubes are available, most of which contain multiple sideholes to prevent tube occlusion. After tube placement, it is important to auscultate over the epigastrium during air insufflation; an auditory "rush" indicates proper tube positioning. Radiographs of the chest or abdomen are also critical to confirm that the tube has been properly positioned before using. On a chest radiograph, the nasogastric tube should have a midline course in the chest, and then deviate slightly to the patient's left as it courses below the diaphragm into the stomach. The tip should be several centimeters below the diaphragm since most nasogastric tubes have multiple sideholes proximal to the tip. Possible complications of NGT insertion are inadvertent intubation of the tracheobronchial tree, esophageal perforation, penetration into the pleural space, or (in at least one rare case) cephalad advancement through the cribiform plate into the anterior cranial fossa. Tubes may also coil or kink in the esophagus or stomach, preventing proper function.

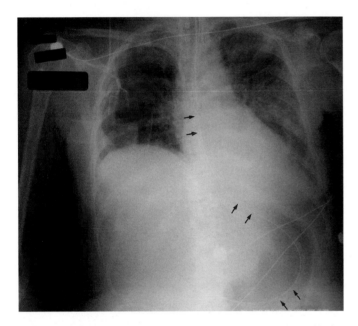

Figure 6–12 Normal nasogastric tube. A transnasally inserted nasogastric tube (black arrows) is positioned through the esophagus and its tip is within the stomach. The gastric air bubble is well seen below the left hemidiaphragm.

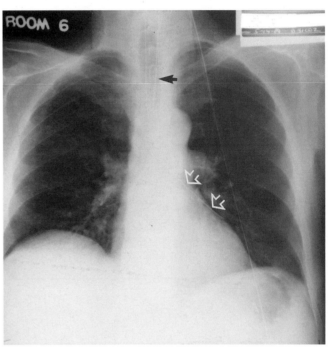

Figure 6–13 Tracheal nasogastric tube intubation. Inadvertent positioning of the tip of a nasogastric tube in the left mainstem bronchus is noted on an AP chest roentgenogram (open arrows). A normally positioned endotracheal tube is also seen above the carina (black arrow).

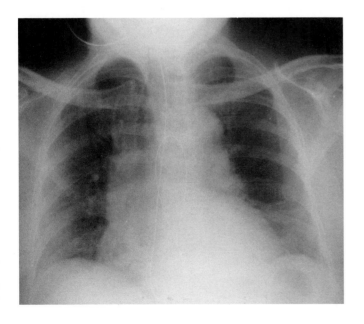

Figure 6–14 Coiled nasogastric tube (NGT). A chest film shows the NGT to be coiled within the esophagus. The tube was subsequently repositioned.

INDEX

161

ISBN 0-8385-4071-6

9 780838 540718

90000

LEE/IMAGING OF THE
ACUTELY ILL